LIVING WITH DIABETES

NICOLE JOHNSON
Miss America 1999

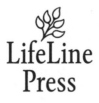

LifeLine
Press

A Regnery Publishing Company • Washington, D.C.

Library of Congress Cataloging-in-Publication Data

Johnson, Nicole.
  Living with Diabetes / Nicole Johnson.
     p. cm.
  ISBN 0-89526-230-4 (alk. paper)
     1. Johnson, Nicole—Health. 2. Diabetes—Patients—United States—Biography. 3. Beauty contestants—United States—Biography. I. Title.

RC660.4 .J64 2001
362.1'96462'0092—dc21
[B]

                                                                              2001038241

Published in the United States by
LifeLine Press
A Regnery Publishing Company
One Massachusetts Avenue, NW
Washington, DC 20001

Visit us at www.lifelinepress.com

Distributed to the trade by
National Book Network
4720-A Boston Way
Lanham, MD 20706

Printed on acid-free paper
Manufactured in the United States of America

10 9 8 7 6 5 4 3 2 1

BOOK DESIGN BY JULIE LAPPEN

Books are available in quantity for promotional or premium use. Write to Director of Special Sales, Regnery Publishing, Inc., One Massachusetts Avenue, NW, Washington, DC 20001, for information on discounts and terms or call (202) 216-0600.

THAT'S LIFE (pp. 199–200)
Words and Music by DEAN KAY, KELLY GORDON
© Copyright 1964 UNIVERSAL-POLYGRAM INTERNATIONAL PUBLISHING, INC. (ASCAP)
International Copyright Secured All Rights Reserverd

I dedicate this book, my heart, to all those affected by diabetes. Your strength is incredible and your determination has taught me so much. Remember, everything in life happens for a reason. I believe we are to use our combined circumstances to effect a change in this world. Together, we can move this mountain of diabetes... we must never give up, we must never stop believing!

All my love and respect,
Nicole

Contents

Prologue

I've written this book for a very special reason. I have diabetes, as do more than ten million other people in this country. Or, to put it more accurately, more than ten million *diagnosed* people in this country. There are over six million others who don't even know they have the disease and who desperately need to be tested and treated. Diabetes, in the words of the Centers for Disease Control, is ballooning into "epidemic" proportions.

But it's a silent epidemic—diabetes is a quiet killer. That's why, as Miss America 1999, I campaigned with the title "Diabetes in America: Unmasking the Hidden Killer." Diabetes kills more people than AIDS and breast cancer combined, but how often—if ever—have you read about the warning signs of diabetes, what you can do to prevent the disease, or what can we all do to cure it?

Chances are, not much. I want to change that.

You don't have to be a medical professional or a scientist to make a difference in diabetes care. I'm not a scientist, and I'm not a doctor. But I think that's an advantage because even though my message is not medical or scientific advice, it's just as important. This is a book about hope and inspiration. This book is about real life with diabetes and the real struggles that accompany this terrible disease. By talking about these issues openly, I hope to help people heal the wounds that often accompany diabetes.

When I was diagnosed, I was a college student, but I had already worked as a professional model, competed in pageants for scholarship money, and had big dreams—not only of becoming Miss America, but also of pursuing a demanding career in journalism. I was a woman who wanted to make her mark on society. And although I didn't know quite how, I wanted to be a catalyst for change. I pray that through this work, you will commit yourself to helping in this mission.

When I was diagnosed with diabetes, I thought my dreams were shattered. I thought my future was over. But it wasn't; actually my life was just beginning.

Diabetes is a terrible disease, but it can be controlled. I am hopeful we will soon find a cure. But the struggle to manage diabetes can also be a universal symbol. We all have obstacles to overcome, we all face adversity in life. Diabetes, for me, was a huge obstacle, but it wasn't the first, nor will it be the last. The universal aspect is that we learn—all of us—through not letting our obstacles impede our path toward success or achievement.

In this book, I want to tell you what it was like to be Miss America—it was both a whirlwind of excitement and, maybe surprisingly, a lot of hard work. But much, much more than that, I want to tell you how I got there, and how I'm carrying on my life's mission today, because the biggest lesson I've learned is that no matter what obstacles life throws in your way, you can achieve your dreams. No matter how lonely you feel—and I've often felt very lonely with this disease—if you keep your dreams alive, you can not only restore yourself, you can do something that's just as important—you can touch others with your gifts.

This is my gift to you—my story, which I hope will both inspire and provide vital information you can use. I pray that God blesses you and touches your life with this story... it is the journey thus far.

Nicole Johnson

PART I: JOURNEY OF A LIFETIME

*"There she is, Miss America 1999,
beginning the journey of a lifetime..."*

Chapter 1

TO BE PERFECT…

To the outside world, beauty pageants are about perfection—a fit body; a sparkling smile; an enhanced evening dress; a flawless talent; a quick, sharp mind; a politically correct answer; a smooth response…perfect poise. Pageants are every bit of what they seem to the outside world…and more. A lot of hard work goes into them.

But if you really want to understand pageants, if you really want to know what it's like to compete, you have to remember that a pageant, any pageant, is a competition between individuals, each with a story all her own. Even greater, however, every pageant is a competition against yourself and your own weaknesses. Pageants are fraught with stories of inevitable disappointments, the courage and dedication to overcome those disappointments, and then the final achievement—for every girl who makes it on stage in a pageant has already proven herself worthy; she's already one of the best.

The behind-the-scenes stories of a pageant can be dramatic. I don't mean the animosities between contestants—I always tried to ignore these. But there's often the voice that feels dry and off-key just moments before a performance, or the girl who pulled a muscle in dance rehearsal who's now called upon to go through a gymnastic routine in front of an expectant audience, the missing gown, the forgotten lines—and judges, those omnipresent beings who are watching everything and who won't tolerate failure.

That is exactly where I was just before Thanksgiving in 1993 as I waited for that final phase of competition at a preliminary competition for the Miss Florida title—Miss Sarasota/Manatee County. Months of work had gone into preparing for this competition. I had strived to combat the weaknesses I perceived in myself. Here, in this pageant, I was in the best position to reach the perfection that I daily tried to achieve. I was used to this sort of pressure, the everyday pressure of competition. I took the nervous tremblings of the flesh in stride; after all, that was just a part of the weakness. You feel the butterflies, you accept the butterflies, you never give in to them.

But what hit me now felt like a deathblow. It was something very, very different from nervous butterflies before a performance. It was a pain I'd never felt before and could never imagine enduring again. It was a pain that felt as if it might rip my life from inside of me—at nineteen, on stage, in a pageant.

"Why is this happening?" That thought ran through my brain, screaming disaster.

I was lying on a wooden bench backstage, holding my abdomen, writhing in agony. I couldn't stand, much less walk. I couldn't even sip water. I felt as if I couldn't breathe—and that meant panic. My mind felt as if it were trembling—and then I collapsed and started losing consciousness. The reprieve from pain would last only as long as I was out and the lapses I was having in consciousness were temporary. After each lapse I would surface again into this incredible agony. It was absolutely terrifying. My body was in rebellion and I was losing control. As a pageant contestant, you're always afraid of losing control. Now I was afraid of losing my life—of blacking out and never coming back.

With just a few hours until curtain, pageant volunteers rushed to find a doctor in the auditorium. When he came backstage, he poked around my stomach and told me my appendix was probably getting ready to rupture. He asked me to do jumping exercises. I thought he was crazy, I couldn't even sit up! But I managed to do as he asked—how I even managed to stand, I'll never know.

"Hmm," he said, examining me as I jumped, and then prodding me again. "Can't say for sure." That is the last I remember of him. I continued trying to get comfortable, but nothing seemed to work. I moved from spot to spot looking for relief, trying to gather the strength to continue with the competition. Later, my parents came backstage, and my mom found me on the floor of the restroom, my head resting on the cool of the tiles—trying to become calm, catch a breath, and wish the pain away.

My parents begged me to leave. I had to see a doctor, they said. But I refused. The pageant would be over in just a few hours. If I could hang in there, if I could overcome this apparent weakness, if I could perform, I might be able to finish the pageant. And if I could be strong enough to overcome this weakness, I might even be able to win. "I've come this far," I pleaded, "...please don't deny me the opportunity to try...."

So there I was, at that final stage of this preliminary competition for the Miss Florida title. How could I not participate? The title was just within my reach. I had been first runner-up so many times. But this time I had worked harder, I had prepared better, I could almost taste the victory. The title...and perfection...were right there, or so I thought.

FEAR AND WONDERING

Yet as I fought to stay in this pageant, I knew something was wrong—desperately, desperately wrong. I tried to push the thought aside—just as I had for a while now. I thought about the last several weeks and, more recently, about this terrifying weekend. For weeks, I hadn't felt right. There had been annoying headaches, dizziness; my eyes were bothering me. I couldn't put my finger on it. At first, I thought that I just needed glasses. But there were other symptoms too. Symptoms I had tried to ignore. I felt extremely fatigued and unquenchably thirsty—all the time, no matter how much water, juice, or soda I drank. Plus I was constantly running to the bathroom. I could have chalked that up to the amount of liquids I was drinking, but I knew that it wasn't normal to get up *several* times in the middle of the night.

So it was more than needing a pair of glasses. I allowed myself to assume that these bizarre symptoms were just side effects from my hectic schedule and busy life. I knew I wasn't eating or sleeping as I should, but who does in college? I was a sophomore at the University of South Florida. In my pursuit of excellence, I wanted to drain every ounce of opportunity from my college days, living them to the fullest—academically, socially, spiritually, and in preparation for a career. So, I carried a full load of coursework, and was involved in everything from music groups to student government—all while holding down a part-time job. I was even president of the Baptist Student Union, the largest group on campus. But for all that activity, and even with some late-night pizza indulgences, I thought I was fit and healthy. No matter how busy I was, I worked out nearly every day.

But even I had to admit something was wrong. I had seen several doctors to find an answer, and I kept following their advice and trying to recover and forget it all. I was a fighter—not a quitter. I wanted to succeed so terribly much. I didn't want to give in to physical weakness—that was one of my worst fears—weakness and failure. This was no temporary fatigue; I'd read somewhere that Margaret Thatcher once said that she got by on four or five hours of sleep a night: it was all a matter of habit and will. But my body wouldn't respond to force of will; it seemed to be rebelling against my habits; but I knew in my heart—I could feel it—that it was much more than that. The symptoms were hanging around like a foul-mouthed and abusive ex-boyfriend. The headaches, fatigue, dehydration, and blurry vision weren't just petty annoyances; they were interfering with my concentration, my schoolwork, and my ability to lead or merely to participate in the groups I'd joined.

On my first visit to the university's health center I was told that I was "probably anemic and should take a multi-vitamin and iron supplements." That didn't work, and I went back to the health center, saw a different doctor, and was diagnosed with the Beijing flu. I was perplexed; I had never heard of the "Beijing" flu. How could I have it—I thought, in my ignorance—when I had never been to China? That doctor prescribed antibiotics, told me to get some rest, and I did feel a little better—I felt well enough, at least, to decide that I wouldn't let a little flu—Beijing or not—keep me down. I pushed myself to go to class. I continued to participate in extracurricular activities. And, yes, on top of all of that, I prepared for the Miss Sarasota/Manatee County competition.

The weekend before Thanksgiving is a busy time for anyone, with the holiday ahead and often more than the usual work to get through. But for me it was also pageant weekend, with the finals on Sunday.

I drove the several hours from Tampa to Sarasota on Saturday morning for rehearsal and the interview portion of the competition. Even though I was again plagued by flu-like symptoms, I was convinced I could still compete, perform, and do it all—and do it all well enough to win. That is, until I woke up on Sunday morning.

I had been miserable all night, but I passed it off as nerves or something I ate, and kept rolling over trying to sleep. But sleep or even rest was evasive. I gave up trying to get some sleep as soon as I could—as soon as morning peeked through the windows—thinking that facing the day would be less frustrating and less exhausting than trying to sleep when sleep wouldn't oblige. I felt a clammy sweat on my body and forehead. Getting dressed was a chore. My muscles ached— almost as though I'd been through a heavy workout. I was fumbling with the buttons on my clothes, when I suddenly had to run to the bathroom, vomiting.

The violence of getting ill left me shaken and in tears. I splashed my face with cold water, gargled, and tried to get a grip on myself. I was still determined to go on, though I knew, at this point, that I needed prayers of support. Coming from a close, faith-based family, I called my parents immediately and asked them to pray for me. They told me I should pull out, that my health was more important than any competition. But there was no way I would quit. I was determined to give my all in the pageant. I remembered what Helen Keller said: "Character cannot be developed in ease and quiet. Only through experience of trial and suffering can the soul be strengthened, vision cleared, ambition inspired and success achieved." For me, this was a character-building moment—I wasn't going to fail the test.

My parents and I stayed in touch by phone the rest of the day; I drove myself to the convention center, cell phone in hand, being consoled by Mom. Driving at this point was no easy task since the pain in my abdomen had grown intense. I would roll down the window to try to get some relief, only to break out in goose pimples and shivers from the fresh air.

Diarrhea had joined vomiting as my twin tormentors—I felt exposed to the possibility of horrible embarrassment. Here I was, on the final day of competition, a day when I should have been limber and confident, and ready to knock myself out to win. Instead I was cradling my abdomen, doubled over in pain, and spending every spare moment in the bathroom, groaning. Even worse, I felt as if I were going to lose consciousness. It was completely unnerving—or not quite completely, because I hadn't lost my will to win. I pushed the negative thoughts as far away from me as I possibly could. I kept gasping, not only for breath, but for the courage to try.

THE SHOW GOES ON

I wanted to keep my game face on, but of course it seemed hopeless. My head was spinning, and my mind kept fading in and out. My ears were scarlet from hearing the girls whispering and gossiping backstage. I was still kneeling on the bathroom floor, and while the bathroom tiles felt cool and comforting, I knew this position made me look as bad as I felt, and the tiles left what looked like a red rash with indentations on my forehead. When I pulled myself upright, it felt as if the room were moving, as if I were losing my balance. I gulped hard to keep another wave of nausea from overtaking me. People around me dabbed my temples with damp paper towels. A hand reached out and supported me by the elbow, and, with quiet resolve, I shuffled to my dressing area.

The opening number was a parade of the contestants—big smiles, good posture; I could not give a sign that I felt worse than I'd ever felt in my life. People often say that pageant contestant smiles are fake—this one was, but I hardly think it could be criticized. The woman who keeps her composure, who smiles when her body is seemingly being ravaged by the worst flu imaginable—to me, that's a good thing. If a beauty pageant is meant to showcase what's best in a woman, I think this is it. It's a kind of strength, a strength that mothers know when they deal with children who are sick and troublesome, and the mother herself is sick, but who has no time—or desire—to think about herself. Pageants can build that kind of character.

Backstage again, I had to change into a swimsuit—about the last thing in the world I felt like doing. A one-piece that clung to my body like a glove was insulting to my aching abdomen. But my name was called, out I went, and luckily I made it back. Then another change of clothes, and I wondered how my lungs would ever find the breath—and I the necessary confidence—to belt out a song while my stomach clenched itself against embarrassment. But I went out there, and, again, I did it.

My appearances on stage felt painfully long, like those dreams you have when time seems to stand still and although you try to run, you don't go anywhere. My only consolation was the backstage bench, where, after each performance, I collapsed and closed my eyes, becoming as still as I could—just a few moments of reprieve that would give me the strength to make my next appearance.

Soon there were only two competitions left: the evening wear, and the on-stage questions. Backstage, they lined us up, getting us ready for our entrance, but I just couldn't go any further. What strength I had mustered to make it this far had gone, I could barely stand, my vision was blurry, and then, incredibly, one of the other contestants, Malina Price, put her arms around my shoulders, her head resting on the side of mine. She softly whispered a prayer, asking God to hold me up, to speak for me, and to heal whatever was wrong. She held my hand as I walked past the curtain—this, too, is the spirit of the pageant, of sister helping sister, a race where there can only be one winner, but where contestants nevertheless support each other.

From her kindness and blessing, I suddenly felt a jolt of energy. I was rejuvenated and through her touch and her prayer I found the new courage to persevere, new strength to support my weak body. I went on stage—I don't remember quite what I did—but I made it. Now I had to do it just one more time; it was time to walk on stage for the announcement of the winners. As we walked out there, I knew I had won...regardless of whose name was called, regardless of who got the crown...my victory was making it to the end! As I was standing there on stage I felt myself swaying, I was getting dizzy again. Malina was standing slightly behind me, and at one point, she had to hold me, literally—and amazingly, covertly—upright. She was my guardian angel.

My name was called as second runner-up. At that point, I was just glad I made it through the pageant—to be called as second runner-up was almost unbelievable. But there was no jumping for joy. Never was I more smilingly sedate—in appearance, anyway—about winning a runner-up position than I was now. I thanked God for letting me get as far as I did. I thanked Him for not letting anything fatal happen to me. I thanked Him for providing me with a friend like Malina.

Chapter 2

DEADLY DIAGNOSIS

After the pageant, my family quickly gathered me into their arms and carried me home to rest. I rationalized that the worst of this crazy flu was behind me and that a trip to the hospital now would be overkill. Home and rest—that's what I needed. I finished taking the flu medication that had been prescribed. But not only did it not work, my symptoms were grotesque. Now that I was at home, not trying to do it all, I became painfully aware of just how sick I was: my hair was falling out in clumps, I was losing weight drastically, and I struggled in the mornings just to get out of bed—the combination of fatigue and illness was almost too much. By now I was willing to do or try anything to stop the excruciating pain.

The day before Thanksgiving, we called every doctor we knew, but no one would see us so close to a holiday—except one, a family friend who arranged to see me at a geriatric hospital that was on his rounds. While I was in the hospital's emergency room the physician did some routine lab work and blood tests and said that although my preliminary symptoms indicated the flu, he would know more after he received the results of the lab work. He ruled out my appendix as the problem and sent me home with a different antibiotic.

The new antibiotic seemed to help, though I still had to go to the bathroom seemingly every fifteen minutes, and Thanksgiving seemed less a celebration than an endurance contest. After the long weekend, and after much debate with my parents about the wisdom of my choice, I went back to school to finish my coursework and prepare for my final exams.

I had been back at school just one day when I received a phone call that changed my life forever. It was Sunday evening, and I was sitting in the dorm room I shared with a roommate. The phone rang and I was glad to hear from Mother. I quickly realized, however, that my father was on the extension. I said hello to him, but he didn't answer. I could hear him sniffling. Suddenly I felt cold and I couldn't seem to breathe; I turned to face my wall as if by doing so I was stepping into a different room, into privacy.

My mother said, "Nicole, the doctor thinks you have diabetes...." The words echoed in my mind: diabetes. "Oh my God, I can't have diabetes." Panic. I can't breathe. Wait, that's crazy! I don't have diabetes. The doctor is wrong. This was even crazier than having the "Beijing flu." I didn't even really know what diabetes was. Wasn't it something that runs in the family? No one in my family had ever had diabetes. The doctor had to be wrong. I heard my mother's voice pierce my thoughts: "Your blood sugar was over 500—509 to be exact—last week. You could have gone into a coma." I didn't know it then, but I would soon find out that a normal blood glucose level is around 100. I was pushing into levels that could be deadly.

But at that moment, I was still trying to wrap my mind around the word. *Diabetes!* A million objections ran through my mind: I'm healthy, I'm too young, I'm ambitious, I have plans—how could God let this happen to me? "Oh my God. Oh my God." I was crying out inside myself for salvation. "God, don't do this to me. Don't leave me here with this terrible disease. God, I don't want to die."

"Whatever you do, Nicole, don't drink any soda. Don't eat anything sweet. We're coming over to get you. We're taking you to the hospital."

My response was immediate and reflexive: "I don't think so! I can't go to the hospital, my exams are right around the corner and I can't afford to miss any school. Plus, there is no way I can leave now, there are planned events this week." Besides, it's all unnecessary, the doctor was WRONG...right, God?

"Nicole, you have to go to the hospital. After that, you'll have to stay at home for a while."

I couldn't agree to that—at least not now—but we reached a compromise. There was a big concert scheduled the next evening and I was part of it. I would perform as planned, the climax of my music class, and then I would let my parents take me to the hospital. I suppose, in a way, it was a replay of the Miss Sarasota County/Miss Manatee pageant: just one more competition, just one more performance, just one more race to run. For all I knew, it might be my last.

Immediately after hanging up the phone, rebellion and anger welled up inside of me. I thought, "No one is going to tell me I can't be like everyone else. And if I'm never going to eat anything sweet again, I'm going to make the most of my last night." As if getting a formal diagnosis controlled how the disease affected my body, I felt invincible until the doctor gave me the final verdict. I decided to salute diabetes by guzzling an entire two-liter bottle of Coca-Cola. Like a drunk saluting tomorrow's sobriety, I lifted the bottle and turned it up. As a final act of rebellion, I refused to use a glass.

If that was crazy—today, it seems even suicidal—it got worse. I knew that if I left school I was going to lose all the meals on my meal card—meals that I'd already paid for—and I was darn well going to get my money's worth. More than that, if the pronouncement of final diagnosis meant giving up sweets forever, I was going to splurge on every sugary dessert I could find. So I went to the cafeteria and gorged myself on food. I had pumpkin pie for lunch, cherry pie for dinner, and Captain Crunch cereal for a snack. At one point I sat and looked at all the food on my tray and broke into sobs.

All I knew about diabetes was that a classmate of mine had died from it in my senior year of high school—for me, the very word diabetes meant death. I had been given a deadly diagnosis. That night, I curled up into a ball and cried myself to sleep. Nothing good was ever going to happen to me again—I had *diabetes*, my life was over.

CONFIRMATION

The next night, I performed at the Civic Center in Tampa. I had worked hard for this concert, and I performed as well as I could. My body, rebelling from the dietary havoc I had subjected it to the previous day, seemed not to be a part of me. At times I thought I would have to sit down on the stage, or I would fall down, having lost my shaky balance. My vision was blurred, and it was impossible for me to read the music.

Later, my parents told me how afraid they'd been during that concert—not knowing if I would collapse, pass out, or even die on stage. They were counting the minutes until they could get me to the hospital.

The entire time I was on stage, performing, my mind wandered. I kept thinking about my future, my horrible, horrible future: needles, tubes, pain, hospitals. *Needles.* That was the worst part. I had always hated needles. When I was a child, it took three adults to hold me down to give me a single shot. I simply could not survive the endless shots of insulin.

When the concert was finally over I felt scared and raw, quite unlike the victory I had felt at the pageant not long before. I didn't enjoy a moment of victory or satisfaction after performing that night. My spirit cried out to God, "Why is this happening to me? Here I am on earth doing everything I'm supposed to do—a good student, a good daughter, a faithful friend, a faithful servant—and this is my reward?" I thought that if God cared, He would stop this from happening. What I would eventually learn was something quite different—I would learn about God's severe mercy, that He teaches us the same way He taught Job and Abraham, by testing our courage, our faith, and our willingness to commit ourselves to service. When my parents showed up at my side, I turned and with quiet acquiescence, I allowed them to take me to the hospital.

The first few hours in the hospital were like something out of a bad movie. I was in denial and I was petrified. I just walked in as if I were checking into a hotel. Only I didn't find myself in a swank hotel room. When I walked into the room, there was no flopping on the bed and flipping through TV channels. Instead I was handed a ventilated gown and told to change in the restroom. I climbed into a bed with white sheets and a thin blanket, if you could call it that. I still remember how cold that room was. And the blanket offered no comfort, no warmth. I wished I had a nice thick comforter that I could pull up to my chin to protect myself from the cold.

Although the nurses and doctors tried to be reassuring, they seemed to be cold as well. All of a sudden, I became nothing but the body that housed me. It was so odd to watch them work on my body as if it didn't belong to me. They even talked as if I wasn't there. Control over my life was completely stripped away along with my shoes and my clothing. I was put in bed and people began fussing over me. A bracelet was put on my wrist, like a handcuff declaring me a prisoner for a crime I hadn't committed. I resented the nurses and doctors who were taking care of me. I felt that they were the ones stealing my life, as if their presence caused the disease. I knew deep inside that it wasn't their fault, of course. It was this monster "diabetes"—it was taking my soul, my dreams, and my goals; it was robbing me of a future. Everyone kept saying that things were going to get so much better for me, but I couldn't hear or understand that. I felt hopeless—and I mean that literally: I felt manacled to this thing called diabetes that thrived on destroying my hope.

I had thrown myself into my college and extracurricular life with enthusiasm because I was eager to succeed, to live life as a high achiever. But now, in a matter of hours, diabetes had pronounced sentence and had crumpled up all my life's dreams and thrown them away, as if they were nothing more than a sheet of wastepaper. I had gone from savoring a busy life of school, pageants, and performances to lying in a hospital bed in a cold, dark, dreary room waiting for someone else, who had more control over my life than I did, to come and stick me with a needle. I was facing a new set of challenges—fear was in session, nightmares had become my reality, and my throat swelled with doubts about my ability to cope. Even though my family was right there and what seemed like a swarm of doctors and nurses hovered around me, I felt utterly desolate and alone.

Then a nurse entered the room and prepared to give me an IV with the insulin and fluids I so desperately needed. But when I saw that IV needle coming at me, my fight-or-flight reflex kicked in—definitely in flight mode. I had put up with enough, I had endured the poking and the prodding; this was getting serious. It was now or never and I was on my way out. My father, who had been by my side the entire time, took one look at my eyes and he knew exactly what I was thinking. Before I knew what he was doing, he quickly grabbed hold of my legs to keep me in place, and when the panic didn't subside, he pinched them as hard as he could to get my mind off the needle. I don't know what hurt more, the needle in my flesh or my father's seeming betrayal of trust. But, just as fast, it was over; the IV was in. My emotions were still running wild; how could my father do that to me? And then it hit me—I could only imagine what the expression on my face had been—I could only imagine what I really thought I would accomplish if I had run out of the room, my hospital gown flapping behind me—the tension burst like a bubble. In the aftermath of what had just happened, what else was there to do but giggle—Mom, Dad, brother Scott, and I.

TAKING BACK MY LIFE

Those first days we were all in a state of shock—maybe bewilderment is a better word—because this new "reality" I had been thrust into was overwhelming. I hated not being able to move around. I hated not being in control of what I could eat. I hated the special meals I was given. They were labeled "diabetic" as if to mock me, and they never included dessert, Coca-Cola, bread, pasta, potatoes—they didn't include anything that I considered normal.

Worst of all, I had to learn to give myself insulin shots—something that seemed on a par with self-mutilation and torture. I hated needles. It was like the ultimate insult. On top of everything else that diabetes meant, I was also going to depend on these needles just to survive. The insulin was just another shackle I had to face. In fact the whole experience was like being held a prisoner: I *lived* in that hospital bed. I hated having to ask for everything. I hated being completely dependent on others.

My desire for independence was very great. I was nineteen, and I had spent the last several years of my life in that teenage battle for independence. I had been fighting for it since high school and was just enjoying the fruits of victory in these first few years at college away from home. Now, in the hospital, my independence was being taken away from me—possibly forever. Or so I thought. In my limited knowledge of this disease a few things were crystal clear: I knew that as a person with diabetes I would always be fragile, always be on medication, always be just one step away from disaster; and in the short term at least, I would have to move back home.

The doctors somberly drilled this into me, telling me that they were doubtful that I'd have the strength to finish college, let alone pursue a career in broadcast journalism. These things—especially my chosen career—were simply too stressful for someone in my condition to consider seriously, they said. If I thought my future was hopeless, the doctors surrounding me confirmed it. Nicole Johnson, Miss High Achiever and Lover of Life, had become Nicole Johnson, diabetic, trapped in a hospital bed. A former beauty pageant contestant, I was now bedecked not by strings of pearls, but by strings of dripping IVs—each drip, a drip of life; each drip, another chain relentlessly tying me to insulin, to dependence on drugs and to other people, to a life, quiet and alone.

I continued my medical education over the next several days. I was instructed on everything from glucose monitoring to mixing insulin to diabetes complications. I received the information reluctantly, because I was exhausted, confused, and angry: this wasn't a subject I wanted to master; it was a subject I wanted to forget.

But I couldn't—and it was frustrating. Many things came easily to me, but I was finding that managing my new condition wasn't going to be one of them. I had to mix two forms of insulin, and I thought, "I'm not a doctor. How can I be expected to do this?" I felt as if I were the only person in the world with diabetes; I had a lot to learn about myself...and about the world.

Everyone said I would feel so much better once I started taking insulin and testing my blood sugars regularly, but I found that life became a lot more difficult. I did get the hang of the daily insulin injections, although I have to admit that I have never really warmed to the idea, and it was difficult learning to gauge when I needed an injection. My blood sugar levels were on a roller coaster—they could be anywhere from the five hundreds to the teens. My emotions followed, and I had zero confidence that I would ever control my diabetes; it was unmistakably in control of me.

It is important to note that diabetes and fluctuating sugar levels cause mood swings. In addition, diabetes can become a psychological battle because of a person's struggle to control something that they never had to think about controlling before. A blood sugar high can make you feel worthless and like a failure because you failed to monitor your condition properly, you ate the wrong thing, you didn't give yourself enough insulin. Lows hurt terribly and make you feel weak, frail, and unable to function. Struggling through the mood swings and the psychological need to be in control left me feeling incredibly vulnerable.

I did, however, have one saving grace. All the nurses on my floor—the ones who assisted me around the clock—were the embodiment of kindness and compassion. It seemed that no matter how moody I became, there was always a nurse nearby with the skills and sensibility to help.

One nurse especially touched me. She was young and upbeat, and I looked forward to seeing her every afternoon. She took time to console and motivate me—her words spoke life to my soul. She made me believe that diabetes wasn't a death sentence; that I could learn to control and manage it; that I *could* live with it. Through this nurse's kindness, I was lifted out of depression and began to see light out of my denial. I told myself that I wanted to help others the way she helped me. Shortly after leaving the hospital, I began to prepare for nursing school taking classes in chemistry and biology. It didn't take long for me to realize that although I was called to help others with diabetes, nursing was not the avenue for me.

My family came to see me every day. They suffered with me during my down times, and although they tried to be strong, they couldn't hide the worry on their faces or the tears in their eyes. Mom and Dad were suffering at least as much as I was; I know that they felt responsible in some way, as parents always do: "Did we give her the gene that caused this disease? Could we have done something different and prevented it?" They were certainly doing all they could now, and I loved them for it.

They were also preparing for my uncertain future. While I lay in that bed and learned all I could about diabetes, my dad and brother moved all of my stuff out of my dorm room and brought it back home. I was forced to drop out of the University of South Florida that semester, because I'd missed too many classes while I was in the hospital, and I couldn't finish the coursework. My new life was about to begin—whether I liked it or not.

BABY STEPS

So, I went home, just as everyone had planned. I didn't give up. In January, I enrolled at the junior college that was just fifteen minutes away from home. Although I felt as if I'd slipped another rung on the ladder of success, it actually turned out to be good thing. I was just beginning to get the hang of this new life, and living at home gave me the time and the help I needed to learn how to care for myself. I started taking classes at the Joslin Diabetes Center in Clearwater, Florida, to learn more about nutrition, exercise, and other lifestyle adjustments important for those with diabetes. Joslin is the leading clinic in the world for diabetes—and the oldest such institution in the United States. Dr. Joslin was one of the first doctors to treat patients with insulin in the 1920s. The main center is in Boston, and the Clearwater center was an affiliate near my home. There

I received the practical instruction to help me face my fears and cope with the new challenges of day-to-day living with diabetes. I also became active in my home church, and the positive people I had around me helped me to gain a true perspective. I realized that having diabetes meant my life would change, but I was gaining confidence that I could *direct* the change. A fire sparked within me—a renewed passion to pursue my goals, to live my life to the fullest. This was MY new life and I didn't want to merely exist with diabetes—I wanted to *live*.

I reached down deep within my soul and gathered up the strength to take each new step toward regaining my life. I was not going to let this monster defeat me. I was going to do everything I could to defeat *it*. My first step in that campaign was when I reenrolled at the University of South Florida in the fall of 1994. I know this was a hard decision for my parents to accept. They felt I needed their protective care, but I knew that I needed independence even more. I had to prove that I could make it on my own—regardless of diabetes.

Brave thoughts, but reality was harsher. I had envisioned life being just the way it had been before, minus feeling sick all the time. But once I got there, I felt alone and depressed because things weren't the same—they couldn't be—and now I was apart from the people who had first fanned the embers of my emotional recovery: my family, my church, and my friends. Again I allowed myself to slip back into resentment; again I was angry with God. I found myself still asking "why" when I should have been asking "how"—how should I live, how could I make the most of the gifts God had given me, how I could use diabetes to help me grow as a person?

The disease seemed so imposing that I wanted to give up— in fact, part of me did. I reached my lowest point when I contemplated suicide as one way of ending the misery that had become my life. It was then that I reached out for help. I sought counseling; I talked to ministers, friends, and family; I asked them to help me stay positive. I asked them to help me as I walked out into this new life. And with their help I pulled through this dark night of the soul, but it was a searing experience, and a sobering one. I learned that I couldn't make it alone—this wasn't a weakness, just a simple confession of fact: no one can make it alone. With the help of those around me, I learned not only to walk with diabetes, I learned how to run. Without realizing it, I had begun to run a new race.

I had thought my life was perfect before I was diagnosed with this disease. I thought that the path I had chosen for myself flowed naturally from my "perfect" world. I came to accept that, as I walked the new path my life had taken, no challenge would ever be final, because life always has new ones. As it says in the Book of Proverbs: "In his heart a man plans his course, but the Lord determines his steps." Challenges can be hindrances or learning experiences. They can be the end of one's life or the beginning. And we each live from one challenge to the next. I could be devastated that the path I chose for myself had been altered, or I could rejoice in the excitement of discovering where this new path was going. It took diabetes to remind me of this fundamental fact of life—and I would soon be reminded of it again, in frightening circumstances.

Chapter 3

OBSTACLES ARE TEMPORARY

I seemed to have beaten the odds and regained control over my life by February 14, 1997. I was living in Virginia Beach, Virginia, in a townhouse with a roommate, and my life seemed to be going reasonably well. I was comfortable with my journalism classes as a graduate student at Regent University and making new friends, enjoying my independence, and generally having a good time. While I still struggled with my diabetes control a bit, that seemed to be par for the course; I was managing to stay away from the extremes, and I was not overly concerned about it. Having just won the Miss Apple Blossom competition, I was in the process of preparing for my first shot at the Miss Virginia title.

Although life was as good as I could hope for, I didn't have a valentine on this Valentine's Day. Considering my hectic schedule, that wasn't surprising, and I celebrated the holiday by going to dinner with a group of girlfriends. There were about five of us and we had a great time as we lamented our universal single status, laughed at the other couples, and just enjoyed each other's company. After dinner we all went back to my house to watch a movie...and that's when things started to change. When we got to the house, I started feeling a little odd—in fact, I quickly became very uncomfortable. I went upstairs, locked myself in the bathroom, feeling woozy and feverish, and then suddenly I vomited. At first, I thought that I had eaten something bad at the restaurant and that it was just an upset stomach. But this pain was far worse. In fact, I hadn't felt anything like it since those days right before I was diagnosed with diabetes.

Fear welled up inside of me. What should I do? After vomiting, what happens to the insulin and the carbohydrate ratio in my body? Am I going to have a blood sugar low or a high? How do I prevent the reaction? What is happening in my body? How do I counteract it? I should have had the answers to these questions, but I couldn't seem to grasp them. I was afraid that this was one of those moments when the diabetes spins out of control and that it was again threatening to steal my life. I hoped I had food poisoning and was merely overreacting, but upstairs, alone in my bathroom, my only companions were pain and fear.

I made my way downstairs and spoke to my friends. Although I tried to vocalize my fears to them, they were uneducated about diabetes and not at all concerned. They advised me to go to bed—which I did—while they stayed up to watch a little more television. An hour or so later, I heard the front door close as they left for the night.

As I lay in bed, I was more worried than I could possibly communicate. I told myself over and over not to panic. It was simple food poisoning. As I chanted that mantra I drifted off to sleep. Unfortunately, I awoke the next morning to even more intense pain and less control over my stomach and intestines than I'd had the night before. I knew something was horribly wrong. I decided I would make it through the day by babying myself—I slept a little longer, ate some soup, dutifully tested my glucose.

The levels were high and creeping higher; as a physiological reaction to illness the liver releases stored glucose. This is typical and happens whenever a person with diabetes even gets a cold. What can be a mere inconvenience to a person without diabetes can lead to fatal results in a person, like me, with diabetes. This was one of the reasons I was so scared. High glucose meant that I was getting closer to a critical situation. But exactly how high was too high in this situation?

Around noon, things got unbearable: I was vomiting, having diarrhea, passing out repeatedly, and my mind felt incoherent. Not knowing what to do or where to turn, I was torn between sheer panic and not wanting to make a scene. I approached my roommate again and tried to express my fear without showing panic. I wanted someone else to make the decision that this was serious, to take the responsibility out of my hands. My roommate still wasn't terribly worried—or helpful. Actually, she didn't seem to pay much attention at all. To me, it seemed that her major concern was her own plans for the day. Since I couldn't stay in my room any longer without going stir crazy, I stumbled downstairs to the living room couch. There, I camped out, trying to rest and watch TV. I thought TV would help me get my mind off myself. I thought I was focusing too much on my symptoms and that I was overreacting.

Early in the afternoon, I was astonished to discover that my roommate had invited friends over to watch TV. In the midst of my obvious illness, they ate pizza and socialized. We all hear of stories about callous people obliviously stepping over some poor epileptic writhing in the street, but I'd never seen that sort of behavior. I was used to being around people who looked out for each other, who had a southern sense of neighborliness and friendliness, who were Good Samaritans. I guess I ought not to have taken that for granted, because these folks could not have cared less that I was sitting there—pale, shaking, and sweating. To them, I was just a bothersome lump on the sofa.

Yes, I felt angry, but pain and illness soon overwhelmed my anger. The smell of greasy tomato sauce, pepperoni, and cheese made my stomach churn, and I had to run upstairs to throw up again. By this time, I was desperate. I called my parents and asked for help, but even as I spoke on the phone, I felt myself fading in and out. I was so fatigued that I literally couldn't keep my eyes open. My mother begged me to call 911, but I was crippled by my fears: I was afraid of giving in to the diabetes, I was afraid of how it would look, I was afraid that I was overreacting and not being sick enough for an ambulance. My mother was afraid, too; she was afraid that I would die while being too stubborn to give in to my fear. She argued with me vehemently. She threatened me. She coaxed me. I finally conceded, not to the ambulance, but to go to the hospital. I called my friend Erin and asked her to drive me there. She agreed, saying she would leave her house in a few minutes to come get me. I prepared to go, but when I went downstairs and told my roommate, she suddenly had a wave of conscience and got upset at *me* for not asking *her* to take me to the hospital. Swaying on my feet as I was, I certainly didn't need another argument. So I got on the phone and told Erin to meet us at the hospital: my roommate insisted on taking me.

At that point, it was obvious even to an outsider that I wasn't doing well. We had to stop the car (my roommate's brand new car; I could feel her grimace) several times so I could vomit. Something was wreaking havoc on my body. When we arrived at the hospital, I went to fill out some paperwork, but before I could finish, I threw up on the nurse. (Now that's one way of being seen quickly in the emergency room on a Saturday afternoon.) I was immediately put in an examining room and, after a few hours, left alone by my roommate, who realized I was going to be there for some time and decided that it would be easier just to come back later and pick me up rather than wait.

I remember sitting alone in the room and wishing I had stuck with the original plan and had Erin bring me. My roommate felt guilty enough to insist on driving me to the hospital, but she didn't realize that I was scared and needed her emotional support more than a taxi service.

What is it about human nature that makes some people insist on being there for the quick fix but not for the long haul? What is it about human nature that makes some people stand by your side throughout any adversity no matter how big or how small? My friend Erin is one of the best, and when she arrived, she decided at once that she would stay all night. I spent hours in that examining room as doctors and nurses came and went giving me exams, blood tests, and more tests. Through it all, Erin stayed.

HOSPITAL NIGHTMARE

I spent most of the time fading in and out of consciousness—or blessedly sleeping. At one point, I was traumatized to realize, through the fog of my consciousness, that I was naked and that the nurses and an attending physician were performing a pelvic exam on me. They hadn't told me they were going to conduct such an exam. They didn't ask my permission; they didn't even let me know what they were about to do. I felt as if someone was invading my body; I wanted to yell and scream but my voice wouldn't come. I was in such a daze, all I could manage were tears that came streaming down my face.

After some of the blood work came back, the doctors called my family in Florida and told them that my body was toxic and my white blood cell count was basically depleted. They weren't sure what was wrong with me, but it was a grave situation and they wanted my parents there as soon as possible. They were preparing my family for the worst.

In the meantime, I had to undergo the most painful procedure I have ever experienced, a spinal tap. They stuck what looked like a horse needle into my spine, and my body went cold as they drew out the spinal fluid. Just like the pelvic exam earlier, the doctors and nurses weren't telling me anything. It was as if my illness automatically gave them control over my body. It was worse than that initial experience I had with diabetes; in that case at least the doctors and nurses were talking to me, explaining the tests and why they were necessary. Here, no one said anything and my thoughts leaped to every disaster in the medical book: did I have spinal meningitis, leukemia, or something equally bad?

Eventually the testing stopped, at least for a little while, and I was moved to a hospital room. My family finally arrived from Florida the next afternoon—I had been in the hospital almost twenty-four hours. When they entered my hospital room, they didn't recognize me. I was having an allergic reaction to the medication the doctors had given me. My face, hands, and body were badly swollen.

On top of everything else, the hospital would not let me see an endocrinologist. To a person with diabetes, the endocrinologist is the specialist who handles everything related to the disease. This whole bizarre episode was doing a number on my diabetes. Yet despite that, the doctors still wouldn't call an endocrinologist. My blood sugar was *way* out of control. I begged for them to at least give me more insulin, but these "professionals" refused. I knew numbers in the high 200s and 300s (a normal reading is between 80 and 120) were not helping my situation, so, I resorted to smuggling in my own insulin and started taking care of the diabetes myself.

The nightmare spun out of control, it was crazy—the doctors and nurses were completely ignoring what I said; it appeared that they knew less about diabetes than I did; even worse, it appeared that they didn't even care. It was beyond belief that they wouldn't give me—despite the fact that they knew of my condition—the amount of insulin that was necessary to keep the diabetes in control. One would think that with whatever else was going wrong with my body, the doctors would do their best not to let the diabetes complicate things. This hospital, if you could call it that, seemed like something out of a surreal Franz Kafka nightmare, where people with diabetes were given invasive strip searches and the most painful medical tests imaginable, but not enough insulin, and not the appropriate treatment.

Even with all of their probing and prodding, the doctors and nurses never determined exactly what was wrong with me. They gave me numerous medications, but they weren't sure what they were actually treating. They finally settled on a diagnosis of salmonella poisoning and gastroenteritis. After several days, I had filled the insurance company's allotted time for that diagnosis and I was sent home under the care of Home Health Nurses. I was glad to leave that hospital— anyone would have been—but I was far from well. My glucose stayed out of control for months after this hospital experience. It felt like all my work over the last few years to obtain control was for naught. It was thrown away and my life was in jeopardy. My risk for complications down the road was increasing with each passing moment.

I still felt very ill, and I had excruciating headaches from the spinal tap, which kept me bedridden in my apartment for several days. According to the insurance company, I was well enough to be home. Yet every day the nurses would come to hydrate me, give me medication, check my vitals, and draw blood. I was also required to make regular trips to the hospital to check in with the doctors and specialists. During that time, I saw neurologists, gastroenterologists, internal medicine specialists, finally an endocrinologist, and the attending physician. During one visit to my attending physician, the unthinkable happened. The doctor, without apparent provocation, turned into a raging lunatic, yelling and screaming at me. He was angry that my family was there with me, questioning him. He yelled that I was an adult and didn't need them there. It was unbelievable; he just kept screaming and screaming and screaming. I recoiled from him, and felt fear and anger. After all, I was the one who had been treated so despicably by this man and this hospital. What more could he possibly want from me? Why shouldn't my parents be there?

I knew from my family and friends that all of the doctors were angry with the number of visitors I had while I was in the hospital. I found out that they were angry at me because I was concerned about my upcoming participation in the Miss

Virginia competition. These health care professionals even criticized my wish to be in the pageant to my family. The most horrible thing was the realization that the doctors seemed to have taken a personal dislike to me—not because of who I was, but because of what I represented. It was a sort of contemptuous, even angry, reverse snobbery: I participated in pageants; I was close to my family; I had the effrontery to treat my own diabetes because they wouldn't—*who did I think I was?* That seemed to be their attitude. *A pretty Miss Goody Two-shoes, with her sweet, little Christian family—and she thinks she can diagnose herself.* I didn't just feel their contempt; it was slapping me in the face.

I simply could not take any more abuse. I was emotionally spent, and I started sobbing uncontrollably. It wasn't the first time I had cried during this latest health crisis. While I was in the hospital I would cry out of sheer frustration because the medical teams would not listen to me. They would not let me tell them what I was feeling or what was going on in my body or that I needed to treat my diabetes—they just didn't want to hear from the patient at all. One of my attending physicians at the hospital even refused to give me my medical records when I asked for them. I don't know if this was just more show of contempt, or if he feared a lawsuit.

I was not only sick, but I was also afraid for my life. The doctors and medical staff failed to follow the cardinal rule of diagnosing—listen to the patient first. Every good doctor I've known has affirmed that basic rule as a key to keeping a patient's diabetes under control. Over the years, open communication with my doctors has provided essential information that has altered my treatment.

But now, at a time when I was so sick, this horrible hospital experience caused me to lose faith in the medical system. I felt physically and mentally abused. Psychologically, I hit a serious low. I felt helpless, tainted, and damaged. And the whole experience made no sense: the violent illness, the near violent treatment, the screaming abuse.

REGENERATING THE ROOTS OF FAITH

In this hour of darkness, I turned to the one thing that had always helped me out of dark places in the past, my faith. I prayed for comfort. I prayed for direction. I felt like a child wandering in circles, lost in a forest. What should I do next? Was I too sick to continue school, to pursue my goals and dreams, to accomplish great things?

Silence.

I felt very alone. I realized that having an illness reveals your true friends—and I had earlier discovered in the course of my struggle with diabetes that most of my "friends" were not friends at all. Now, after this latest health battle, I discovered again that many of those people I had surrounded myself with were merely "fair weather friends" who withdrew from my life while I was in the hospital. Between my roommate, the doctors at the hospital, and my insurance company, I got a quick and nasty education about how uncaring people can be, and about how so much is decided by what is expedient, rather than what is right. At the same time, I realized that each of us is blessed with only a handful of genuine, loyal friends in life, and I was thankful for those friends that stood by me during this time of trial. Shortly after I began to recover, I resolved to adopt a new outlook. I knew I needed to meet some new people; I needed to be closer to God. I needed to be exposed to more in life. Every one of these needs brought me to a single idea: I needed to get more involved in my church. So one Saturday night, I decided to go by myself to a church concert.

It was good to be there alone. I was less inhibited. I was able to worship God without worrying what my companions would think. I wasn't distracted. I lost myself in the music and the message of hope, restoration, and resolve. I asked God to show me His plan and purpose for my life. I accepted the possibility that diabetes would always be a part of who I am. I asked Him to somehow turn this horrible disease into something positive. As I asked for His direction, I was also asking for the confidence that I knew could only come from Him.

The next morning I was awakened by the answer to my prayer. I awoke to a vision of comfort and compassion. I was at home in my apartment, when I heard deep within my heart what seemed to be a command to be still and wait. I wasn't sure if what I heard was my imagination or if I was still dreaming, but I found myself obeying that simple command. Within moments, in my mind's eye I saw a young woman lying in a hospital bed. There was a doctor in the room—and a presence. I say *presence* because it wasn't really a human being—it was in the form of a person but it was surrounded by light.

Nothing like this had ever happened to me before. I was awake—I wasn't dreaming. I wasn't near death; this wasn't a near-death experience. I was fine. I'd recovered. And as shocking as this vision was, I wasn't afraid. I continued to sit... still and silent.

I had a sense that this presence was sweet, comforting, and peaceful. It held my hand and told me everything was going to be fine; the presence took my hand and the doctor's hand. "I will never leave you or forsake you. . . . I began a great work in you and I will be faithful in completing it."

I did not hear the words, but they came vividly to mind. I don't know how often prayers are answered with a vision, but I felt that mine had been. I was changed in that instant. I received reassurance from the Lord. I received guidance.

With the Lord's reassurance and with His guidance, came a knowing. I know as certainly as I know anything that when modern medicine falls short or the human body seems mysterious, there is a wisdom that surpasses human intelligence. There is room for the miraculous. There is room for divine intervention. Why does God let certain things happen? Why does He allow obstacles to seemingly block the path? Perhaps it is so that we can grow in wisdom and learn to help others. As it says in the Book of Isaiah, "For I am the Lord your God who takes hold of your right hand and says to you, do not fear; I will help you."

The whole dreadful experience at the hospital made me sensitive to the difficulties so many people face in getting proper personal care in the impersonal setting of a modern hospital. It's an attitude that I've since vowed—on behalf of other people with diabetes—to fight wherever I can. This is a disease about *people*, not about making it easy for doctors and insurance companies to file forms. Ironically, two years later when I was Miss America, this very hospital gave me the opportunity to fight such abuse when it asked me to speak at a local event! I accepted, and was glad to speak about treating patients as people. I gave them an earful about the need for doctors to listen to their patients, as well as to treat them with proper respect and compassion. Patients aren't just numbers, they consist of so much more; they are *individuals*. To be a good physician, one must treat not only the perceived illness, but also the heart and mind.

LIVING WITH FAITH—AND SEEKING ACCEPTANCE

When I received the devastating news that I was afflicted with Type I diabetes, I was only nineteen. At nineteen, that news became a huge, seemingly insurmountable obstacle in my path. Obviously, dealing with a disease is a physical challenge, but as I had seen in my own life, it is much more than that. It is a mental and spiritual challenge as well. We must learn to accept ourselves, admit that we need help, and embark on our personal journeys of healing. That journey needs direction— and direction comes from the goal. And it comes from knowing that the goal, if more distant, is still possible to realize.

In a book of inspirational quotes, I found the following anonymous description of overcoming obstacles, a quote I have always drawn strength from.

> The sea is dangerous and its storms terrible but these obstacles have never been sufficient reason to remain ashore...unlike the mediocre, intrepid spirits seek victory over those things that seem impossible...it is with an iron will that they embark on the most daring of all endeavors...to meet the shadowy future without fear and conquer the unknown.

From tragedy to triumph, from desperation to realization, I learned that diabetes did not have to conquer me. Despite a severe medical condition, despite the sometimes harsh and dismissive opinions of others, I knew I could achieve my goals, if only I could find the source of my strength.

Having obstacles to overcome is common in all of our lives. I am no different. But I know one thing has made all the difference for me—my faith. It pulled me through this experience—it is as necessary to my life as my insulin—and I cannot talk about Nicole Johnson without revealing the Love of my life and the Source of my very being. My faith has helped me overcome and succeed in spite of every obstacle I've ever faced. Now I recognize diabetes not as a roadblock to the path I have chosen, but as an obstacle that can, through faith, be overcome.

This faith that I use on a daily basis to help me overcome these obstacles is an old friend to me. I was fortunate enough to know faith from a very young age—actually it was the biggest part of my life while growing up. It was a good thing, too, because I have had opportunities to exercise that faith from early on.

I went to Northside Christian, a private school in St. Petersburg, Florida, until the seventh grade. In the eighth grade I switched to a public school, an experience that changed my life. For the first time I had to learn the value of self-respect. At Northside, I had been with a group of kids from the beginning of school. We were more like brothers and sisters than like ordinary school children. The kids were generally nice to each other and came from relatively quiet, sheltered backgrounds. Not that we didn't know how to get in trouble from time to time, but the trouble I was used to was the kind that is spawned from rambunctious play and childhood squabbles. In the public school, the kids seemed a lot more negative, perhaps because they were exposed to many more harmful influences at young ages. In this environment I was not only challenged with having to make new friends, I was now in a place where views were different. I had to learn who I was, what I wanted to stand for, and whom I wanted to stand with.

Like most young people, all my life I've wanted desperately to be accepted—to be part of the best group or the "in" crowd, to be popular. As an eighth grader and a new teenager, I was almost desperate for that acceptance. At the public school, I never quite achieved it; I always felt a bit different, a bit of an outcast. I had the uncomfortable, awkward feeling of not quite fitting in—in any situation. I didn't understand why this was so. Even though I had struggled with this need to be accepted at Northside, it had never felt like such a big deal before. "Besides," I thought, "I am a nice person, I am attractive. Nothing sticks out in the wrong place." I couldn't put my finger on anything that catty prepubescent girls could make fun of. Still, I couldn't get into that inner circle.

So you can imagine how excited I was when I received an invitation to another young girl's birthday party at my new school. I was absolutely beaming. Someone actually thought enough of me to send me an invitation. Maybe I wasn't such an outsider after all. But when I got to the party, it didn't take long for me to realize that this wasn't an "in crowd" that I wanted to be a part of. I assumed this party would be like other birthday parties I'd been to—cake and ice cream, giggling and laughing, games and opening presents. But this party was different: first, there were boys and girls at this party; second, there were no parents at this party. The only chaperones were the birthday girl's older sister and her boyfriend, hippie wannabes, who smuggled in some beer, hard liquor, and cigarettes, and decided that, instead of "pin the tail on the donkey," drinking games and smoking would be the evening's entertainment.

I had to decide: Do I stay and finally achieve that goal of acceptance? Do I do what I know in my heart is wrong? Or do I go home and risk being rejected by these people I so desperately wanted to fit in with? Full of hesitancy and uncertainty, not wanting anyone to notice my fear, or the tears that I could feel pooling in my eyes, I called my parents and asked them to take me home.

Monday at school the word was out: Nicole left the party. Nicole was a goody-goody. Nicole didn't want to have fun. My little thirteen-year-old pride was crushed. Had I made the wrong choice? But looking back I realized that was an important learning experience—I learned what it was like to be set apart. I survived the scrutiny. It was okay to be different. I learned what it meant to listen to that still, small voice that's inside each and every one of us, the voice that whispers in our ears and tells us which way to walk. I had to learn to trust that voice. Thank God that I did. If I hadn't, perhaps I would truly have been all alone, without even faith to help me through when I was diagnosed with diabetes. Perhaps, rather than fighting to succeed I would simply have given up. One thing is for sure, if I had made a different choice that night I would have regretted it for the rest of my life.

I went to high school with that same group of kids, always feeling as if I didn't fit in, always wondering about the future, and always praying that God would send me someone I could trust and with whom I could have fun. God did answer my prayers, eventually. But this was a time of testing. I have only a few close friends from that period in my life. All my social interactions, my roots, were developed or grounded through involvement in my church.

For my family, going to church was not just going to church. It was a way of life. It was our sustenance. I was six years old when I truly understood what I had been learning about Jesus as a toddler in Sunday school and at chapel at Northside Christian. That night, saying my prayers with my mom, I wanted to know exactly how He could live in my heart. As a young child, I made a commitment to live for Him. When I was thirteen, when I had reached an age where I could be held accountable for my decisions, I was confronted with the choice between His way and my so-called friends' way. It was then that I recommitted myself to search for the right path and follow it.

MORE CHOICES

Not every challenge to faith is as straightforward as the party and the peer pressure I faced that night as a young teenager. Some are more subtle. Some find you when you think you are on the right path. It was not much later that I had the opportunity to fulfill a "dream come true" for a young teenage girl.

"Have you ever thought about being a model?" a woman asked me while I was shopping in the mall one day. I looked around to make sure she was talking to me. To my delight, she was.

Now, I don't care who you are, deep down *every* young girl has dreamed about being a cover girl or a supermodel. Despite my conservative upbringing, I was no different. My eyes brightened and I looked at my mom, seeking her approval. We took the woman's card; she ran a modeling agency. Before long, I found myself attending her school to acquire the necessary polish, meeting with photographers, and before I knew it I was actually signed on as a professional model! The agency was a subsidiary of Elite modeling in New York, the home to supermodels like Cindy Crawford and others.

I was even sent to Tokyo, Japan, for the entire summer after my junior year of high school. What an incredible experience: I was an international model! What could be better? This was my reward for walking the straight and narrow! I went by myself and lived in an apartment that housed two other young models. My roommates changed from time to time—and they came from all over the world—but they all had one thing in common: they were wild! Drugs, alcohol, smoking, sex—you name it, they dabbled in it and it was offered to me. But, thankfully, I was strong enough to say no. Again, while it wasn't an easy decision to make, saying no came with less of a struggle this time around—while I wanted to fit in, I wasn't willing to pay so great a price to do so.

For me, this was a chance to do something I'd always wanted to do; it gave me a kick-start onto a possible career path and a chance to save money for college. No desire to fit in was going to compromise my faith or my position with the agency. Ironically, I was eventually "let go" by the agency when I turned down a lucrative job that required me to pose nude. After I returned from Japan, the agency had asked me to consider dropping out of high school and do modeling work that included nudity. At eighteen, with college looming before me, I made the decision that ended my modeling "career." There are times when you have to stand up for your beliefs, no matter what it may cost you. This was one of those times, because without the money I could make from modeling, finances would be tight during my college years.

PURSUING EDUCATION

Unlike most teenagers in high school, I was obsessed about planning for my future. I would go to the library and spend hours researching universities and resources for scholarships. I knew money was tight for my family, so I made it a point to find scholarships. In my research, I discovered that the Miss

America program was the largest source of scholarships for women in the world. I made a mental note to apply once I became eligible as a senior in high school.

Coincidentally, during my senior year, I discovered that the local pageant for Miss Seminole was going to be held in my own high school auditorium. I entered the competition with enthusiasm—my eyes were focused on the scholarship money—but I couldn't help but get excited by the glamour of it all. This was even more exciting than modeling had been. I looked forward to being on stage, dressing up in an evening gown, and performing in front of people. So I mustered up the nerve, participated all the way through, and was named first runner-up! I was shocked! Most of the girls who competed were the popular ones I had idolized for years. I couldn't believe my fortune. Now I was bitten by the pageant bug! As shocked as I was at making it that far, I remember thinking, "What could I have done to push me over the top? What could I have done to get those few extra points to win the title?" My heart was committed. I wanted to compete again. I wanted to improve myself. I wanted to earn the scholarship money.

A few weeks later, I entered the Miss Polk County competition and placed as a finalist. This competition was larger and was open to any girl in the state. I was enthralled with being involved in a big production that was choreographed with music and lights. It was an escape for me—and even a form of corporate acceptance. There was a very practical side to this too—I succeeded at earning enough money in each competition to help fund the tuition costs for my first semester of college. Another obstacle down.

UNIVERSITIES AND PAGEANTS

Cobblestone walkways, white columns, a sense of history, and ivy. I was simply enchanted by Stetson University, a private school with a top reputation in my home state of Florida. I was eager and ready to start. This was going to be a new life. *My* life. A chance to learn, a chance to mature, a chance to grow.

University life exceeded all of my expectations. I immediately began making new friends. I had a serious boyfriend for the first time. I got involved in everything from religious organizations to student government. I was even elected president of the student union board—unprecedented for a freshman woman. My confidence soared. But while I was basking in the glory of these achievements, my life started to unravel on another level. I was feeling run down, very tired (even lightheaded and dizzy), and I was losing a great deal of weight. But I kept my health concerns to myself. I thought by acknowledging them I would somehow make them worse. It's bad psychology, I know.

Throughout this time I continued to participate in local pageants both to satisfy my cravings for a title and for scholarship money. Ultimately, I was gearing myself up for a chance at the Miss Florida title.

Before now, I hadn't given my platform—that is, the advocacy or the community service issue I had to choose as a pageant contestant—much thought. One of my many extracurricular activities at Stetson was encouraging children to read. Every Wednesday at 3:00 P.M. I would go to the local elementary and middle schools in the area and read together with the children. I also spent time tutoring a young girl in fourth grade. I decided that this was my passion and a worthy cause for a pageant contestant—literacy and children. This was the cause I wanted to make my own.

So with literacy as my platform, I competed in three or four other local pageants that year. First runner-up, second runner-up, first runner-up—I placed in all of the pageants, but I never won. It was great to place, but disappointing not to win—especially because I couldn't figure out what was holding me back, what I needed to change. I sought advice from others who told me I needed to lose weight (even though I was very thin). I was told to change my talent, which was singing. But if my voice couldn't carry me through, I didn't know what would; my high school choir director had been one of my pageant mentors. I was told to sharpen my interview by boning up on current events. All of this advice was like encouraging me to change myself. It all seemed impossible. But I worked at it and continued to try. The advice was helpful in many respects—I learned more about myself and who I wanted to be. Looking back on it now, I know that this was all just part of the process of "growing up."

Pageant standards are, of course, measures of perfection. No one can be as perfect as the ideal woman that the world is constantly yearning for. But I was trying as hard as I could to be that perfect person. Perhaps trying *too* hard; in a sense the pageant competitions only reinforced my own perfectionist tendencies. It took me years to recognize that the pressure of always trying to appear perfect held me back from revealing my vulnerable side—even to close friends. But I learned that friendship is all about sharing—vulnerability as well as strength.

Toward the end of my first year at Stetson I received another disappointment, another obstacle to impede my goals. My academic scholarships had been cancelled for reasons I didn't understand. I had done nothing wrong. I had done well academically. But the scholarships had evaporated— evidently some budget cuts for financial aid at the university. I couldn't afford to go to Stetson without that academic scholarship assistance. Neither my family nor I could make up the financial shortfall. Winning money in competitions was not sure enough—just because I had been a finalist several times didn't mean I could do it again. So I made the tough decision to move back to the Tampa area and enroll at the University of South Florida. I would have done anything to stay at Stetson. My year there was one of the happiest of my life. It was everything I had ever dreamed college would be. Now it was gone.

In contrast to the beauty of Stetson, the next fall, I moved into a grungy, cinderblock dorm at the University of South Florida. I had a roommate, but I didn't have many friends. I didn't look forward to starting the process all over again. All I had was my zeal for education and achievement. I wanted to see things happen. I wanted to find my path to the future, my purpose in life. But it was then that my world came crashing down with the diagnosis of diabetes. Again I had been given an opportunity to face another obstacle and to see what faith could do.

Chapter 4

CALLED FOR A PURPOSE

"Girl in the green sweater, please step into the aisle." I had my eyes closed and didn't realize the minister was talking to me until someone caught my attention. I moved to the aisle as he asked, nervous and not knowing what to expect.

I was attending a church service with my parents in Clearwater. It was soon after I had reenrolled at the University of South Florida, and although I was still struggling with my diabetes, I had a new resolve. I was determined not to let defeatist feelings get the better of me; I had decided to reach out to others to pull me through this time of trial. I turned consciously to my faith to sustain and support me. The service had already begun when I arrived. In fact, it was only a coincidence that I was even there; my classes had been canceled that evening and I took advantage of the unexpected break to meet my parents at church.

Now, standing in the aisle, the minister, Reverend Joey Hipp, started talking about a dark cloud that had been over my life. He said, "You think the cloud is so dark that you will never see light again; you feel that God has deserted you." I had been crying out to the Lord for help, he said, and had felt as if He had abandoned me.

"God is with you—so close that you can't see Him," he told me. I began to shake and cry. How could this man know so much about me? "You will find favor with judges, and one day God will put you in a high position to help many people.... He has heard your prayers for a godly husband, and He is preparing this man for you. Do not be afraid. God has heard the desires of your heart."

At this moment I knew his prophecy was real. *No one* knew that I had prayed for my future husband for years. And his words about the "dark cloud" were equally true. I had been careful to acknowledge God publicly just as I always had, but in my heart, every time I prayed I wondered if God was really with me. Because I questioned God's presence, I felt as if His light was missing from my life. I had actually felt several times over the last few months as if I was walking around under a dark cloud. My life had seemed to me so fragile and my spirit so restless. But as I made my way back to my seat, my heart was filled—for the first time in months—with hope. I was stunned that I had been chosen, and that God had spoken to me through this minister. When I drove back to my apartment that evening and contemplated the words that were said over me, I was tingling with a sense that I had been a part of something inexplicable—and true. I thought of something else—of finding a pattern in my life, of trying to decipher God's plan. I had been nursing thoughts of going to law school. When the minister spoke of judges, is this what he meant? More deeply, I began to reflect on my disease, to remember that throughout the Bible, throughout life, it was suffering that seemed to be the most profound teacher, for Moses, for Job, for so many. Without a test, there is no testimony. Perhaps diabetes was my test. I now definitely saw it as shaping my own testimony.

This prophecy had given me comfort and reassurance. It was God's way of reminding me that He was still with me. It also caused me to reflect on where I could make my greatest contribution to other people. Before, competing in pageants, I had had to develop a platform issue, and, looking among my extracurricular activities, I had settled on child literacy as the most important. But that had been a choice, and in some ways an abstract choice given that I did not have children of my own. Now I was *living* a platform issue. Now I had the passion—and the authority—that comes from personal experience. I decided to use my disease to preach the virtues of preventive medicine, of testing for diabetes, and embracing a healthy lifestyle that might prevent the spread of the most common Type II diabetes, and would control the complications of the rarer Type I variety. Armed with my new platform, I reentered the Miss Seminole pageant in the spring of 1994, and, this time, for the first time, as if in proof of the validity of my new platform, I was the winner.

Success is contagious. As Miss Seminole I made my first bid for the Miss Florida title and won the swimsuit competition (even though I wasn't the skinniest girl on stage!). The next spring I succeeded again when I became Miss Florida State Fair. Oddly enough, the future Miss America 1997, Tara Dawn Holland, was my predecessor and crowned me that evening. It was for the Miss Florida State Fair competition that I helped create the "Fair Bear." Fair Bear and I would go to schools and teach children about healthy eating habits. Along with the Fair Bear program, I created a program called "F.U.N. Fitness," which stood for Families Understanding Nutrition and Fitness. The idea was to teach children about the importance of starting early with exercise and healthy eating. I took another stab at the Miss Florida title and placed in the top ten (closer!). I went on to win the Miss University of South Florida title the next year, in 1996.

On my third try at the Miss Florida title, I hit another obstacle. My hopes were high, and I honestly thought the third time would be the charm. Actually, because I had just graduated from college and put my life on hold to go to the competition that year, I *expected* to win. I was even receiving more positive feedback than criticism—which was a new experience. But when the top ten were called, I wasn't one of them. My string of victories had halted; my momentum stopped short. Looking back, I realize that failure, too, can be a positive experience, in that it builds character and helps one appreciate success all the more when it comes. I would later learn the truth of what Booker T. Washington said long ago: "Success is to be measured not so much by the position that one has reached in life as by the obstacles which he has overcome while trying to succeed."

But now I was a graduate without a job. I was still looking to fulfill that prophecy, to do something for God. To me, that meant further education: if I was going to do something about this disease, I had to be properly prepared and trained. God had given me gifts; He had given me the opportunity to speak to adversity and see results. I owed it to God, if not to myself, to do my best with what I had been given. Just as in the parable of the talents, I would be judged on whether I had put my particular gifts, no matter what they were, to the best possible use.

FINDING A HOME AND WINNING THE PRIZE

"This girl belongs here at this school." That's what Dr. Slosser, one of the founding professors of Regent University, said to me as he grabbed my hand and my mother's hand. I was so proud to hear that. Regent was everything I wanted: a graduate school with an outstanding program in broadcast journalism—indeed, with practical, real world experience available right next door at CBN (Christian Broadcasting Network)—a Christian philosophy, and an old Virginia architectural atmosphere. It felt like the perfect fit. My plan was to pursue a master's degree in journalism and then, maybe, go on to law school. Regent was everything I was looking for in a university; this would be a new start.

I worked hard at my studies and accepted that my pageant days were behind me. My education would give me the tools necessary to fight diabetes and succeed professionally. I was absorbed in my classes, but occasionally I'd be reminded—somewhat against my will—that there were still other dreams I might want to pursue at the same time, other ways that I could earn scholarship money, other ways to serve a worthy cause. I don't think I ever really let go of the idea that if I could win a state pageant I would have the necessary vehicle to *really* promote diabetes awareness.

One night during class at Regent, Amber Medlin Ufkes, a former Miss Virginia, leaned over and whispered, "Nicole, I dare you to enter the Miss Apple Blossom pageant. You really should do it. You've been in pageants before. That was my title a few years ago."

"Amber, I really don't want to do it. Pageant life is in my past. That kind of thing is over in my life."

Amber is a very persistent woman. Over time, she convinced me to enter the Miss Apple Blossom pageant. To be honest, I still felt burned-out from losing Miss Florida three times. But the Miss Apple Blossom pageant is an important one in Virginia. It has a reputation of grooming strong contenders for the Miss Virginia title. Eventually I felt myself rising to accept the challenge. I entered the contest, trained for it, and on a cold, snowy night in Winchester, Virginia, I won! This meant I was back in the business of competing. Having won Miss Apple Blossom, I was automatically set to compete in the 1997 Miss Virginia pageant.

I also had more opportunities to get involved with the local and state chapters of the American Diabetes Association. I gave speeches, was appointed to a state legislative coalition on diabetes issues, and went all out promoting diabetes awareness. My goal was to be more than a beauty queen; I was going to make a difference.

AN INSULIN WHAT?

At one of the local ADA meetings, I met sales reps for a company that distributes insulin pumps. It was the first time I had heard about such a device. I was fascinated. I asked question after question. How could a device that looks like nothing more than a simple pager do what took me several shots a day to accomplish? I was amazed. On a visit to my health team, I confided to my nurse that I wasn't doing as well as I wanted with my diabetes—the four to five shots a day really weren't working well. It was at this time that I first spoke to a nurse about the insulin pump. As a result of our conversation, she suggested something that would forever alter my life, a trial run on the pump. On a Friday afternoon in April, I went to my local diabetes clinic in Virginia Beach, Virginia, to try out a test pump for the weekend. I was excited and nervous at the same time. Part of me wanted to prove that I could break it, that it would fail me, that it really was too good to be true, that I didn't need it, but another part of me was fascinated by the technology and seduced by the promise of freedom and flexibility.

Because exercising is one of my favorite pastimes, one of my first tests for the little device was a trip to the gym. I worked out for a very long time—longer than usual—with John, my workout partner and a dear friend. I remember that as we left the gym, we began having a theological discussion about medicine and healing and faith. We were so engrossed in this conversation that when we got to the car we just sat there talking for more than an hour. John listened, supportively, as I raised all my fears and concerns about using the pump: If I wear the pump, does that mean I'm giving up on God and saying that diabetes has won? Am I admitting failure? Does it ruin my chance of ever being considered normal? What will people think when they see it? What will my future husband think? By allowing me to talk these things out, John helped me to see that my concerns were small matters compared to doing what was necessary for my health. Friends who are willing to listen with understanding hearts are extremely important in times of uncertainty. It was so refreshing to be able to unload all my fears and frustrations without having to worry that my friend would be offended. Without judgment, John helped me to accept that I could both believe in God's healing power *and* use the best available medical technology.

Eventually, the pump would be my liberation, but at the time, I could only think of it as yet another defeat. If I took the pump, it meant that I had failed to control the disease on my own; from now on I would have this *thing* attached to me; there would be no way to hide that I had diabetes. I didn't want the pump. I wanted a miracle instead. But because I couldn't break it, because it did everything it was supposed to do, because it really would help control my diabetes, I relented and ordered one. I knew I needed answers and help. Maybe this was the miracle I had been looking for.

Three days before I left for the Miss Virginia competition in Roanoke, the box with my insulin pump arrived. I felt simultaneously thrilled and remorseful, and terribly afraid. It wasn't until that afternoon that I even opened the box. My pageant director, Elaine Aikens, and I decided that we would take the pump out and try it on. The pump looked like your average pager, small, square, and black. I remember I was wearing a white pantsuit and I lifted the vest and attached the pump to my waistband. I saw the expression on Elaine's face and knew that the pump was obvious. I ran upstairs and looked in the mirror. All I saw was this dark bulge on my waist. You could *see* it. I had been told that it wouldn't be noticeable. I had been told that no one would have to know I was wearing it. But there it was. It looked twice as big as it had in the box, and with this white pantsuit there was no way to hide it. I went to my bedroom and cried.

But I was getting ready for the Miss Virginia pageant and I wasn't going to let anything bring me down. Nothing was going to stand between me and this competition. And a huge black pump hanging off my waist would certainly do that. (The pump actually weighed only 3.5 ounces, less than a quarter of a pound, and it was only about 2 by 3.4 inches. But to my reeling mind, it weighed five pounds and was the size of a small purse.) Who wears a pager on stage? And that is exactly what everyone would think I was doing. I put the pump back in the box. That was it, I wasn't going to wear it. I wasn't even going to think about it. I did not want it to dampen my spirits.

I was so excited about going to the pageant that even during the preparations for it, I felt as if I were starting over. I felt I had been given a second chance. I felt that I was in control of everything. I was the captain of my own ship. I was focused. I knew what I had to do. But I still felt the pressure of competition. Only two Miss Apple Blossoms in the pageant's entire history had failed to make it to the Miss Virginia top ten. I sure didn't want to be the third.

I did well in the early competitions and was feeling very good about my chances as we approached the finals, which were two days away. Elaine and I were sharing a room at the Hotel Roanoke and Conference Center. Everything was going well and I was feeling confident. Tomorrow would be the day before my talent competition day. I knew that I needed as much rest as possible, but again my plans were scuttled. During the middle of the night something terrible happened. I had a severe insulin reaction (no one knows why they happen, and I certainly don't know why I had one that night). The next morning around 5 A.M., Elaine woke to find me unconscious on the floor of the bedroom. To this day, I have no memory of getting out of bed, but somehow I did and was able to wake Elaine before I collapsed. Elaine must have been terrified. She immediately called my parents—who were staying in the same hotel—for help. Thank God they had come up to watch me compete in the pageant, as they usually did. If they hadn't been there, who knows what might have happened to me.

According to my parents, by the time they arrived Elaine's face was a picture of fear, for she knew that my coma-like state meant I was in grave danger. My parents started pouring Coke and orange juice down my throat—anything they could find to raise my blood sugar. Everyone was so frantic that even simple things became complex. They couldn't work my blood glucose monitor. Finally they just slashed my finger and dropped blood onto a test strip. My blood sugar was so low it didn't even register on the monitor. (That means my glucose was below twenty points or twenty milligrams per deciliter. At a blood sugar of forty you start losing brain cells.) My pupils were dilated, and I couldn't see clearly. I wasn't able to move my arms or legs or feel my extremities. After seeing no change in my condition they called 911. My mom, with tears streaming down her face, put her arms under mine, picked me up off the floor, held me tight, kissed me, and started praying— "Please God, don't make me lose my daughter." When she stopped praying, I opened my eyes and my first words were, "Mom, does anybody know?"

My greatest fear was that people would think badly of me, that I would lose my chance to become Miss Virginia, that because of this disease I would lose my chance to achieve *anything*. I was terrified of being "labeled." I was terrified of people thinking that I was not capable of doing things. I didn't want to be kept out of any activity. I didn't want to be kept from participating because of diabetes. I didn't want diabetes to ruin my life. I felt at the time that my diabetes had already taken so much away from me. When you have a chronic disease, you feel tainted, you feel like damaged goods. I felt that way. That's why I was trying to keep it private. That's why the issue of the pump being slightly visible was so traumatic for me. I know it sounds ironic because of the platform I had chosen, but I had managed to keep my platform and my personal life separate to a certain extent. My platform was about education; it was about others, not about me. I was about to realize that I would never succeed at what I was trying to accomplish while trying to hide my personal battle against diabetes.

So much for wanting to keep my diabetes private! The paramedics arrived with a stretcher and started running tests. They didn't take me to the hospital and I didn't go to the doctor. This was just as breakfast was being served to all of the Miss Virginia contestants. In my hallway just outside my door, people were standing there with plates of scrambled eggs—gawking, whispering.

I was told to drop out of the competition. I refused. I was determined to prove that I could do it—insulin reaction or not. Once I got the sugar I needed into my system, I slowly returned to normal, if you can call it that. The swing between highs and lows wreaks havoc on the body; I needed rest and missed most of the morning rehearsals, but I was back and ready to go by lunchtime. That night I went on stage and performed my heart out even though my body felt frail. The themes of the song, "With One Look" from the Broadway play *Sunset Boulevard*, were incredibly apt for my situation: it was all about vindication, not giving up, remaining yourself in the face of all the odds. Many have told me it was one of the best performances of my life. Even so, after everybody knew about my episode, I didn't think I had any chance at all. Of course, I was bombarded with questions about my diabetes, which I felt was a defeat in itself, having hoped that it would not even be brought up. But when the final night came around, I was named number ten of the top ten. That's as far as I got, but that was okay with me. I had done it. I had been a finalist in a state pageant—even while recovering from an insulin reaction. I felt a curse over my life had been broken. My failures in the Miss Florida competition were behind me.

Sure, there were naysayers. Someone even approached me after the pageant and said, "Don't ever do this again. You'll never win. You'll never be Miss Virginia because of what's wrong with you." The sad thing is that, for a while, I believed that advice and let such negative voices resonate in my heart and mind. For a short time, I gave in to their cynicism. Today, I regret every minute that I listened to those without faith, hope, and confidence. What they didn't realize—and what I was about to find out—was that there isn't a perfect mold that we all fit in. The beauty of life is the diversity that surrounds us. The challenge of life is to fulfill your dreams.

After that terrifying insulin reaction, I knew I couldn't give up on my diabetes or my hopes and dreams. As Michael Jordan once said, "I expect failure—everybody fails—what I can't accept is giving up." Within days, I decided that I needed to use the most aggressive therapy available. In my heart, I knew I had to take the pump out of the closet and put it on my body.

It was one of the best decisions of my life, a decision I wish I had made long before.

With the pump, a weight had been lifted. I felt like a person again! When I was diagnosed with diabetes I realized how many things I had taken for granted. I had taken for granted simple decision-making abilities: when to sleep, when to eat, when to wake up, what to wear, when to exercise, and how much I could do in a day. Now, through this tiny little device, which sent insulin into my body in regular intervals much like my pancreas would if it worked properly, those decision-making abilities were given back to me. The tremendous freedom and flexibility outweighed its small inconveniences. The pump gave me the most beautiful gift I could ever have been given: the opportunity to see a dawn every morning and a sunset every evening, the opportunity to live again.

With my renewed spirit, I decided to ignore the advice I received after that last pageant and I pursued the title of Miss Virginia one more time. My platform would be the same, only this time it would be stronger, this time I was going to be the real Nicole Johnson—with diabetes, with no regrets, with nothing hidden. I realized that I had been through an incredible process over the last several years. Although I had struggled to squelch the striving for perfection, and just do my best, I had never really gotten away from wanting to be the perfect woman. Trying to hide my diabetes had almost cost me my life. I had to learn that being a person with diabetes is nothing to be ashamed of. Now, with the pump, I vowed to compete again, and do my best to see that people were educated about diabetes: not because it was my platform, but because it is my life and because there are more than sixteen million people across the United States with the same condition . . . many unaware . . . most embarrassed . . . all needing a voice.

You can compete in the Miss America system for six years, from the age of eighteen to twenty-four—that's it. I had started participating when I was eighteen. I was now twenty-four. This was my last chance. I intended to make the most of it—insulin pump and all.

Chapter 5

COMPETING WITH HOPE

To qualify for Miss Virginia and have a chance to win Miss America, I needed to win another local title. I decided to try for Miss Lynchburg, which, like the Miss Apple Blossom pageant, was one of the premier contests in the state, with an equally good record of launching Miss Virginias. The Miss Lynchburg pageant had the additional advantage of offering a $1,000 scholarship as well as a clothing stipend for the Miss Virginia competition—both of which I needed. At the time, I was working two jobs just to make ends meet.

The Miss Lynchburg pageant lived up to its reputation and was one of the most competitive contests I'd been in. One of the contestants was even the first runner-up from the last Miss Virginia pageant. I looked at my fellow contestants and was convinced that my chances of winning were pretty slim. As the runners up were announced, the tension mounted, and I felt breathless. It was one of the most nerve-racking moments of my career. This pageant was my last chance at Miss Virginia and therefore my last chance at Miss America. So much rested on what the judges decided, and as I stood there, looking at the other contestants, I couldn't believe they'd decide in my favor. The other girls were far more talented than I was, they were more beautiful, and they had more personality. Any one of them would have been a wonderful representative for Lynchburg. I stood there and prayed. I prayed they would call my name—and when they did, I was both stunned and ecstatic. I know that some people like to dismiss the emotions of beauty pageants as being somehow plastic or artificial, but no joy was more authentic than mine when I surprised myself by winning the Miss Lynchburg title. I felt my future blooming with hope and opportunity—and also a new resolve. As I prepared for the Miss Virginia pageant, I decided I didn't want to hide behind a platform of preventive medicine, preventive health care, or my F.U.N. fitness program. My platform would be diabetes awareness, and I would be completely open about my condition, my life, and my experience.

I threw myself into the cause, increasing my volunteer work with the American Diabetes Association, writing stories for diabetes websites, and participating in various diabetes events in five states. I also became involved in the Lynchburg community. In the three months between Miss Lynchburg and Miss Virginia, I was always on the go. Usually, given that so much of it was diabetes work, it was rewarding and enjoyable. Sometimes, though, I saw what life could be like when it moved too fast.

I traveled to New York City on a shopping expedition with the Miss Lynchburg committee that was preparing me for the

Miss Virginia pageant. It was a fun trip, but I found myself in some uncomfortable situations. It was almost like being back in school. I didn't fit in with the New York City nightlife of drinking, foul language, and sexual innuendoes. Sitting in a smoke-filled bar, listening to people talk about their sex lives, and hearing their lewd commentary on everyone who walked by made me think I was in the wrong place. At one point, I excused myself from the restaurant and went back to my hotel alone. I felt guilty for ducking out like that, and I certainly didn't want my friends to say that I was being holier-than-thou. But had I stayed, I would have felt worse.

The experience in New York was educational in another way. Traveling with the Miss Lynchburg committee made me begin to appreciate that if I did indeed win Miss Virginia—and later, Miss America—I would have to get used to being shuttled around by "handlers." For someone who valued her independence, this was an unnerving thought. As it turned out, I didn't know the half of it.

Preparing for Miss Virginia itself was a monumental task—and a real character builder. I faced personality conflicts, wardrobe issues, and even controversy about my talent. You name it, it happened! I was told that I was fat. I was even ridiculed by my preparation crew—in front of other people! I was lectured about my talent. Statements like "Lose that vibrato!" or "You just shouldn't sing that song!" were just some of the "constructive criticisms" I heard several times. Although this was nothing I didn't expect after four previous state competitions—three times in Florida and once in Virginia—the criticisms always hurt. To be honest, as the competition approached, I was getting weary of the verbal sniping, endless workouts, and headaches that come from trying to please everyone. I was a little older than many of the girls, and had simply outgrown a lot of what was going on. I tried my best to ignore the gossip and focus on the competition.

Miss Virginia is a weeklong event, beginning with interviews on Tuesday and Wednesday. Preliminary competitions take place on Thursday and Friday night, with the final competition on Saturday. For me, the competition began with a few minor glitches. The first problem was that I arrived at the competition without a talent costume. Well, that's not exactly true. I had an outfit. Unfortunately, it was this horrible Middle Eastern costume that made me look like Barbara Eden in *I Dream of Jeannie*—just not as cute; and in my opinion, since no one can match Barbara Eden, these costumes should be retired, much like a football jersey number. In any event, it was really awful, and I was mortified to think that I might have to go on stage looking like that. Thank God some good friends found an outfit for me at a formal shop in the area. The loaner outfit was perfect. It was red, it looked great, and I felt great in it. One glitch taken care of.

The other problem was that the dress for my opening number didn't fit right—it had only arrived the day I left for Miss Virginia, and we hadn't had time to fix it then. So, it ended up being a work in progress all week. It was completed just a day before the stage presentations—just one more glitch to overcome. Still, as far as my health went, I felt great—and that was the most important thing.

As the week progressed, the competitive atmosphere moved into full swing, with gossip and egos so ridiculous that it was actually funny. For instance, some girls tried to predict the winner based on who would look best in the Miss Virginia prize car. One mother loudly announced that she and her daughter had already booked hotel rooms in Atlantic City for the Miss America competition. I noticed that some people were practically obsessive about their preparations, their gossiping, and their sniping at each other. I ignored it as best I could, trying to stay focused, calm, and peaceful, but it is hard in such a stressful, emotionally charged atmosphere— especially when much of the gossip is about you.

Some of the contestants, as well as others, were buzzing about my diabetes. Their stories were so negative and full of misinformation that they were practically public service spots about the need for diabetes education. I was actually accused of faking my diabetes to gain an advantage on the other contestants. Some took another tack. One person, referring to my dressing glitches, said, "Well, what they're saying must be true—that you have some kind of disease—because so many things are going wrong for you." That was so catty and ridiculous that I could easily laugh it off. But the gossip and catty statements also made me more determined to win. I told myself that I could do it, that Miss Virginia (and ultimately Miss America) is about more than crowns and cars. I vowed to myself that I would show them—and the doctors who had told me I'd never do it—that a person with diabetes could compete and win.

I especially looked forward to the interview competition. It wasn't that I wanted to win it so much as that I wanted to get my point across about diabetes awareness and how we need to do a great deal more to confront this deadly disease. Part of the interview competition takes place offstage, early in the week. It's a chance for the judges to go in-depth with the contestants, and that's the interview I was most interested in. In the offstage interview you have more time to really share your heart. By contrast, in the on-stage interview, which happens during the evening gown competition, your answers have to be short. I wanted to inspire the judges with my conviction that diabetes education, testing, and research is a cause that needs our urgent and dedicated support. I had the zeal of a convert when it came to diabetes awareness. I had the personal experience from being someone who ignored the warning signs of diabetes—increased thirst, urination, and fatigue—and almost died because of it. I wanted to help other people with diabetes, I wanted to motivate everyone else to help people with diabetes, most of all I wanted to motivate those judges to help me help others.

My interview went well, and by the end of the week there were two clear front-runners—Nita Booth and I. As I stood on stage, one of two finalists, I remember praying, just praying, that the dream would continue, that I might win and have another opportunity to gain an even bigger, national stage for my cause. As I looked at Nita, I saw an incredible contestant; in fact, I could think of only two advantages I might have. First, I was older, which might give me an edge in maturity as a spokeswoman. Second, I had my cause; I had a mission, a burning passion within my heart, to help Virginians by educating them about diabetes.

When my name was called, I was electrified with joy—joy at victory and opportunity realized. I was going to the Miss America competition. After five years of seriously competing in pageants, I was going to the biggest pageant of them all, representing the state of Virginia, whose history, traditions, and people I had come to love. I always knew that Virginia would be my home. When I was eleven years old, I went to Virginia for the first time on vacation with my family. We went to Virginia to experience its history—and I still have the

"Virginia Is for Lovers" bumper sticker that I got on that trip. Although I loved growing up in Florida, the history and the beauty of the Commonwealth fascinated me. It was amazing to realize that in Virginia I could literally follow in the footsteps of such American heroes as Thomas Jefferson, George Washington, and George Mason. What a legacy, what a history, what a place to live!

Victory in hand, I could not rest—and I mean that literally. Though I stayed at the exquisite Miss Virginia suite at the Hotel Roanoke and Conference Center the first week after the pageant, I got no rest. I was too busy that week with meetings, paperwork, and more meetings, and through it all, even when I tried to rest, my mind was constantly racing with ideas of what more I should be doing. Even without sleep, I had a great time—it was one of the most hope-filled and anticipation-filled times in my life.

It wasn't all giggles and strawberries, though. I made the very difficult decision to confront the Miss Virginia Board with my concerns about the backstage atmosphere of the pageant. I told the board that they needed to do something to end the nasty bad-mouthing and bad behavior I had seen among the girls and other people involved in the pageant. I reminded the board of their responsibility to ensure that girls were treated respectfully and that the social atmosphere did not become poisonous backstage and during the preparation for the competition. It was a very hard thing to say—because I was so grateful for having won. But I felt I had to do it. I did not want other girls—especially girls battling diabetes or some other affliction—to have to go through the hurtful gossip and put-downs that I had gone through. The Miss Virginia competition should be above that, and I'm hopeful that today it is.

MISS VIRGINIA ON PARADE

As Miss Virginia, I rode in a few small town parades, attended local fairs, and enjoyed my first blitz of media exposure. At each event, at every microphone, I advocated fervently on behalf of people with diabetes, diabetes research, and education. Early in my term, *The 700 Club* TV show did a story about my struggle with diabetes. It was a terrific honor; the reporters did a very detailed story, and the national exposure it gave to diabetes awareness was very rewarding to me. It was the first taste of what newfound celebrity might achieve for the cause of diabetes awareness. Articles began to appear in newspapers as far away as Texas about my journey thus far and my desire to educate people about diabetes.

While all of my appearances as Miss Virginia were wonderful, one particularly stands out in my memory. I was scheduled to give a concert as part of an ice cream social at a retirement home in southwest Virginia. I was shocked to be greeted by reporters, television cameras, and crowds of people—all of whom wanted to talk about diabetes. The reporters wanted to hear my story. The people wanted to tell me their own stories about friends or loved ones who had been stricken with the disease. Most of all, they came to encourage me. I couldn't help but cry—not tears of sadness but tears of gratitude. Never before had I so connected with an audience in talking about diabetes. Never before had I felt such overwhelming kindness from a crowd. Never before had I felt so close to others who were suffering. The words of Psalm 10:17 seemed appropriate: "You hear, O Lord, the desire of the afflicted; you encourage them, and you listen to their cry."

What I remember most about that afternoon was not the attention, nor the standing ovation; it was a precious gift given to me by a paralyzed man in the audience. He had drawn a picture—with his teeth—of me singing. His drawing—and his courage—reminded me that challenges and obstacles are to be surmounted, precisely so that we can give ourselves to others. I met many people with that same spirit, during my time as Miss Virginia, including Ben Meyers, a radio host who had overcome homelessness. In fact, meeting people of this caliber—heroes who surmount challenges—was probably the most important thing I experienced as Miss Virginia. When you meet so many brave people, some of it can't help but rub off—and I found that Virginia was full of brave, gracious, and friendly people. I was honored to represent them.

The honor also came with a heavy responsibility. My next stage would be national. The Miss America pageant was quickly approaching and would be held in September. That competition would be my third in barely six months. Never would the pressure be greater. This was my last chance to be handed a national platform for my cause. The odds of becoming the next Miss America seemed much smaller than one in fifty-one. And yet there I was, one of fifty-one women, representing the Commonwealth of Virginia, representing all those people I had come to love since winning the crown.

THE NATIONAL STAGE

The Miss America pageant stretched over more than two weeks, and although the actual pageant is held in Atlantic City, the first four days were spent in Orlando, Florida. Those four days were extremely busy. There were photo sessions, videotaping sessions, a film shoot on a Disney cruise ship, a parade on the Walt Disney World boardwalk.

On the third day, the six finalists for the Quality of Life award, which recognizes community service, were announced. When my name was called as one of those finalists, I literally jumped for joy. Simply being recognized as a finalist was a tremendous validation of my work for diabetes awareness. Not long ago, I had been ashamed of my condition and tried to hide it—courting death rather than admit I was a diabetic. Now, because I'd used my affliction to help others—many of whom were suffering far, far worse than I was—I was making a difference in the world. I had always wanted to do something important. Now an esteemed American institution that provides more than thirty million dollars of scholarship money every year was giving me recognition for doing just that. I felt as though I was finally beginning to achieve my goals. The competition ahead began to look like an added bonus. I asked God for the grace and the ability to touch even more lives.

Those four action-filled days and late nights in Orlando took their toll. I think every one of the girls was exhausted when we said goodbye to Disney World. From Orlando, we flew to Atlantic City—a flight I'd heard a lot about because many girls fall apart at this point. As I watched the girls around me, feeling exhausted and excited, I understood why this day is so tough for competitors. Everyone is tired and in that time when there is no agenda other than the trip, the girls, for the first time, have the opportunity to think about the pageant ahead. They realize that they are on the verge of the biggest competition of their lives, their chance to become Miss America, and all of a sudden the pressure is too much for them to handle. You really start to feel the intensity of the competition, and for many girls it is overwhelming. I noticed the tension as soon as we boarded the plane. You could see it on the faces of the girls, in their movements, and in some of the things they said—criticisms, calculations, speculating about who might win. Some girls actually dealt with the pressure by counting themselves out, resigning themselves to the notion that others were better. But no matter what happened, we all realized that in eleven days one, and only one, of us would be crowned Miss America 1999.

When we got to Atlantic City the frenzy of the previous four days returned with a vengeance. As soon as we got off the plane, we were ushered into a wild press conference. The continuous barrage of flashbulbs and the hollering of reporters were overwhelming—every imaginable news organization was there.

With that press conference, I was thrust back into the competition. I sought reactions from others—and hoped for, and generally received, praise. But I also sought—and kicked myself when I drew—criticism. Each of us had a few moments to speak in front of the group—a daunting experience, knowing that this would be the crucial first impression we'd make with the press. I thought that I did well. I felt sure that I had made a good impression and been confident, convincing, well spoken, and well received. In usual competition style, I sought the professional opinion of Margaret, my pageant traveling companion. A loquacious southern blonde who would herself have made a formidable opponent in her prime, Margaret had been involved in pageants for almost twenty years, and I deferred to her experience frequently. In this case, she let me know the deflating truth: I could have done better.

Although being back in hypercritical competition mode could be disheartening, I quickly shook off my disappointment and proceeded enthusiastically to the next step. I was in the Miss America pageant! I found myself relishing every moment—knowing this experience would be full of lasting memories. The media attention was flattering, and I was elated when a photographer took a picture of my insulin pump, something that at this pageant I was proud to advertise.

Of course, the excitement of the pageant was coupled with hard work. There was less than two weeks to learn the dance routines, to be fitted for costumes, and to have our shoes inspected. Shoe inspections are conducted because contest guidelines include a heel height requirement. I ended up as one of twenty girls whose shoes were too tall. Mine were over the standard by half an inch. It never feels good to be singled out as a rule breaker, but it is even worse to suddenly need new shoes when virtually every hour is scheduled with rehearsals, interviews, and all of the other events.

One morning, in the midst of that week of rehearsals, Margaret woke me with screams of joy. My picture was on the front page of the local newspaper, the *Atlantic City Press*. It accompanied a story about my wearing an insulin pump. Surprisingly, several girls approached me after reading the story and apologized for being unfriendly. I was so busy trying to master the dance routine, worrying about finding new shoes, and trying to find time for everything else I had to do that I hadn't really noticed getting the cold shoulder from any of the girls. They thought my pump was a pager and that I was trying to say, "I'm a big shot. I'm so important I have to wear my pager *all* the time." When they learned that it was an insulin pump, they were mortified. Their apologies meant so much to me. I know it takes courage to admit you were think- ing ill of someone, and even more courage to admit it to that person. It was a good feeling to have their respect—especially since I was beginning to think that this was another one of those environments where I just didn't fit in.

The next big step for me was the interview that would help the judges select a winner from the six finalists for the Quality of Life award. The interview was held about ten days before the finals—when Miss America would be named! I found myself sitting at a huge rectangular table with the panel of judges. We discussed the relevance of my platform to corporate executives, children, teens, parents, the elderly, and others. I was thrilled to feel as if we were having a conversation, not an interview. In many ways, it felt as if I were defending a dissertation. What I remember vividly, though, was that the new Miss America Organization CEO, Rob Beck, was sitting in the back of the room, listening in. At one point, I looked over at him and saw tears streaming down his face. In that moment, I knew my message was getting across. I had come to this pageant—not simply for a title—but to make a difference. Rob Beck's tears were proof my goal would be realized and my prayers had been answered.

After the Quality of Life interview, I was even more eager for my favorite part of any pageant competition—the offstage interview with the judges. This interview was the most important of my life—it would determine my future course. The air conditioning in the room was so cold—and the wait so impossibly long—that I did jumping jacks and stretched, just to keep my blood flowing. It sounds funny, doing calisthenics as I waited, but everyone seemed to have a silly little ritual they performed to ease the tension.

I remember sitting in that cold, sparsely decorated room waiting for my turn. I was aware of the significance, felt the stress, but I also felt at peace. So many of the things that had happened to me in the last five years were culminating in this moment. My platform was an issue I cared about more deeply and passionately than I could have ever imagined before I had diabetes. It was no accident that I had come to this point not when I was younger, not when I was free of this disease, but now. It is written in Psalm 27, "Wait for the Lord; be strong and take heart and wait for the Lord!" God had determined my fate up to this point. I would trust Him now as well.

I remember the other girls. I saw them pacing, cramming, rehearsing, even reading several newspapers at once. I didn't think there was anything to be gained by that kind of cramming. I'm sure I wouldn't have absorbed anything that way even if I tried. Instead, I said silent prayers, asking God to keep my heart at peace and my mind focused.

Finally, it was my turn. I remember standing in the hallway, rehearsing my key points and my mission statement. I knew exactly what I wanted to say. The interview started slowly—the judges themselves seemed nervous—but then the conversation flowed and even became emotional. Several judges wiped away tears as we talked about the challenges of diabetes, how I had felt close to death, how committed I was now to teaching people about treatment and finding a cure. I felt my words were getting through. And then it was over. My heart was pounding so hard I could hear it thumping in my ears. When I found Margaret outside, a dam of emotion burst in me. We jumped and screamed and held onto each other and sobbed, but they were tears of accomplishment. I had drained myself in that interview. I had tried so hard to express my feelings—feelings that were as real as the cold bathroom floor I'd collapsed on years ago, as real as the children I'd met who were already

facing a life of insulin shots—and doing so with brave, coura-
geous little smiles. Once you have diabetes, a whole other
world opens up to you, a world of hidden heroes overcoming
a sometimes grievous pain. I wanted the judges to know about
that world, to know that it was a world inhabited by millions of
Americans. I tried. I think I succeeded. I know that after the
tears I felt exhilarated and happy.

Chapter 6

SHOWTIME

The rehearsals continued right up to the opening night. With each day the rehearsals seemed more intense. Girls began to show the strain, which was understandable. This was by far the most stressful pageant environment I had seen. We were committed to preparing for this pageant twenty-four hours a day. So when opening night came, it was a relief. But there was also an electrifying sense of excitement. This was it. It was finally real.

DAY ONE

Music exploded from the orchestra—it was "There She Is, Miss America" played to a modern beat. We heard the pounding applause from the live audience, and I felt myself choking with emotion. I was so busy praying for calm that I nearly forgot I had to get out there and dance. The dance routine was followed by the famous parade of states. I was sure that in the excitement I would forget, but luckily I did remember to look for the Virginia delegation in the audience. I was grateful for everyone who'd made the sacrifice of time and money to come cheer for me. Part of me wanted to run over to them so we could share the excitement together.

The night went well. I made it through the evening wear competition without tripping over my train. I had tripped over my train a few times in rehearsals, and I had been afraid that I would do it again. I walked, I turned, I answered my question, something about successful women, and finished my appearance without incident. Thank goodness! With that, two phases of the competition—and the evening—were finished. The remaining events would be completed over the next three days. I made my way back to my room and crawled into bed, with a mixture of joy, relief, exhaustion, and dread of the remaining competitions.

That dread was well founded. My worst recurring nightmare was about to rear its ugly head.

DAY TWO

The next day, I felt sick and almost fell during rehearsals. The nurse noticed that my balance was off, but when we checked, my glucose levels were fine. What was happening? I felt miserable and my head was pounding. When I stood up the room would spin.

I spent most of the morning resting in the nurse's station. As I lay there, my mind flashed to other pageants, other disasters. I couldn't believe that having come all this way, I was going to be struck down again. But here I was, lying on a cot. Wondering if my body was going to forsake me again. I pleaded silently, "Not again, please God, not again!"

While I rested, the other contestants practiced for the swimsuit competition. I needed the practice. I had never been on the mechanical rotating stand—which I imagined would be the *perfect* thing for someone feeling dizzy. I needed the extra practice walking in the new shoes I would be wearing, and I was nervous about the swimsuit portion of the competition in general.

The swimsuit competition has always been the hardest part of pageants for me. In preparing for both Miss Virginia and Miss America, I was never able to diet because of my diabetes. Unlike the other contestants, I couldn't go on some carbohydrate-free crash diet or overdo it on the workouts to drop pounds. My goal for this competition wasn't to be skinny, but to be physically fit at a healthy, normal weight. I knew that I had achieved that. My trouble now was being strong enough to stand up. I don't think anyone really relishes the idea of standing on a stage in a swimsuit and high heels for everyone to judge her body. But let me tell you, it's even harder when your eyes are seeing spirals, your head is pounding, and you're worried about throwing up on stage. I can honestly say that the one thing I will not miss about pageant life is standing in a swimsuit on a runway. At the same time, I do believe the swimsuit competition is a vital part of the Miss America pageant. I am totally opposed to those who want to do away with it because it's supposed to be "sexist." The swimsuit competition is central to the tradition of Miss America. The pageant began as a swimsuit competition more than eighty years ago. Today, the swimsuit competition is worth only 15 percent of the scoring, but it does give contestants a chance to demonstrate their personal pride, discipline, and good health. And because good health is something that I advocate, I support the swimsuit competition.

At that moment, though, *recovering* my good health was my primary concern. By the afternoon, I started to feel better and was able to rejoin rehearsals. Even though my initial concern was about my diabetes, sometimes my prescribed daily medication gives me headaches, and the nurse and I finally attributed my problems to a severe migraine. All I really needed was that morning's rest—and having gotten it, disaster was averted.

That night the audience was rowdier and even larger than the night before. People were waving signs, banners, and even lights. The swimsuit competition went well. I wobbled a bit on the rotating platform, but I didn't fall off—and after the morning's fright, that seemed like a victory. When the evening was over, I felt that the last fourteen days of nonstop action had truly worn me out. But as is the custom, after each night, the girls have the opportunity to visit with their state's delegation. I looked forward to my time with family, friends, and supporters. So, although I was tired, it was another night of tumbling into bed far later than my body would have liked.

DAY THREE

The next day was talent day. I spent the morning rehearsing, but I still felt tired. I had diverted it for a while, but the stress I had seen on some of the other girls' faces had finally gotten to me, too. I was a full five pounds lighter than when I arrived in Orlando two weeks before. As a result, my talent outfit was too big. During rehearsals, I showboated like a comedian for my supporters in the auditorium by holding my pants out in front of me. I could stretch them out so far I looked like a walking— or singing—commercial for some weight loss program.

Next to the swimsuit competition, the nerves I get before the talent competition place a close second. I've never been confident about my singing—at least in front of judges (in church, I have no trouble at all). Here I was at the Miss America pageant and these judges were the best. I was really nervous that night. I gave it my best shot, but when I walked off the stage, I was convinced that I had lost. I just wasn't good enough, and I wished I had a second chance. But that was it. The next stage of the competition was the announcement of the top ten finalists on Saturday. I didn't need anyone else's opinion to tell me that I had blown this one. For me, the competition was over. It was a horrible feeling.

All I could do now was wait for the announcement of the top ten finalists. That was almost forty-eight hours away—which seemed, at the time, like an eternity. I knew that there were people waiting for me just like the last two evenings. I hurried to my assigned area, looking for a familiar face. Even as my supporters crowded into the area, I couldn't retain my composure any longer. I was scared, filled with doubt, and emotionally spent. It had been the longest two and a half weeks of my life. I remember collapsing into my mom's arms. It was as if she and I were the only two people there. I cried little girl tears that only a mother can handle and became a sobbing puddle, but I had to pull myself together. So many people had come to see me. The area was filled to capacity with aunts and uncles, directors from past pageants, the whole Virginia crew, old coaches and acquaintances, even people I didn't know. Everyone was smiling. They didn't think I had just lost. They were all so encouraging and gave me such a boost. My parents told me that I had done a terrific job. My brother leaned over and whispered, "Nicole, I really think you could win this thing. I've never heard you sing so well." It was such a wonderful thing to say; I took him at his word. Even though I still had some doubts, his words began to renew my confidence.

A DAY OF WAITING . . . AND PREPARING

The next day, Friday, was stressful. The contestants were all on edge. There were still more rehearsals for the final show. But everyone was exhausted. When the girls weren't dancing, they collapsed. The place was littered with sleeping bodies— on dressing tables, on the floor, under the tables, curled up in corners. No longer did we carry books or newspapers to the convention hall—the item of choice was now a pillow.

We had one more official event before the following night's show: a parade down the famous Atlantic City boardwalk. The boardwalk is where the Miss America pageant began in 1921. The parade each year has become a part of the history and tradition of the pageant. As we stepped into the vehicles we would ride in the parade, each girl became a part of this American tradition. I rode in a convertible and was decked out in jewels to accent my black velvet and synthetic fur gown, and princess slippers—outlandish shoes are a tradition of the parade. As I rode down the boardwalk, people were yelling all kinds of encouraging things, but the one that I heard the most was, "We've picked you as the winner!" At first I was stunned and then flattered. That was great—and so was seeing the Virginia state delegation with their official Nicole T-shirts: "We're here to *pump* you up!" And then there were all the kids with diabetes waving signs.

My heart swelled with emotion, and I had to fight back tears that threatened to slide down my cheeks. As far as I was concerned this parade was for them. These children were the reason I was there. Our shared experience made us vulnerable and determined. And I think they knew that at this pageant I was competing for *them*. We shared the same hopes and dreams. If I won, I would have a platform that would educate the country about their plight. I vowed again that they would be my priority.

THE BIG MOMENT

The next morning, we all stumbled into the convention hall at a painfully early hour—given that we knew we'd be kept there until after midnight. It was going to be a *very* long day. We worked hard to ensure that this final night of competition, when the television cameras were rolling, would be perfect. That meant rehearsals and more rehearsals.

But then it was time. Our backstage room buzzed with local hostesses, contestants, production staff, and Miss America officials. Everybody was focused on the coming production. We were all also sadly aware our time together was almost over. We would soon be saying goodbye to people we had practically lived with for weeks; or perhaps, as we got swept up in the post-pageant chaos, we might not even have a chance to say goodbye. Many staffers asked us to sign their program books as souvenirs, and girls exchanged addresses. I remember a few of the ladies from the staff grabbing my shoulders and telling me how nice it was to work with me. I looked them in the eye and told them from the bottom of my heart that the pleasure was mine. They had been awesome to work with. They had done their jobs with joy. They had been so helpful.

I spent that evening running back and forth to the bathroom. It wasn't a problem with the diabetes, I knew. I was just dealing with those ever constant butterflies that accompany you to these competitions. This time, the symptoms were almost welcome. This was it. I was at the final stage of competition. I had seen this night again and again on television. I had watched the beautiful women. This time I was one of them.

After what must have been my fifth trip to the restroom, the contestants were called to the stage. It was just a few minutes until the curtain went up. Several of us took a moment to pray together, to share our faith: I was honored to be among these women. In those last few moments before we went on stage, I thanked the Lord for such an incredible experience.

Then the music started. We performed the opening number, which was followed by the Parade of States. The crowd went nuts—and I loved every minute of it. The Virginia group was crazy—I could see them jumping, clapping, giving me the thumbs up sign. Some of them were crying! It was as if they already knew I had made it to the top ten.

As I ran off the stage to change, something inside of me gave me pause. I heard a voice in my soul say, "Rest, for you have done all you needed to do, I am in control and your life will never be the same again." As I walked onto the stage to get in place for the announcing of the Top Ten, I, too, started to cry. There had been a lot of tears these last two weeks, but I knew that no matter what happened next, this had been the greatest experience of my life. I was forever changed. The cameras flicked on, the music started, the crowd screamed, and they began to call the names. "And our first Top Ten finalist is...Miss Virginia, Nicole Johnson!"

The crowd exploded. I ran, jumped, and beamed. What an honor, what joy. The vision of my family and friends celebrating in their seats will be forever a part of me. The rest of the finalists were called. Of the ten, I could not have picked the winner. For that matter, I could not even have picked the Top Ten. I stood there with the other finalists when I suddenly realized what was going to happen next. It was the swimsuit competition, and I was going to be the first contestant on stage. The cameras went to a commercial, and I remember beginning to politely wait for the other girls to walk off the stage. Many were just frozen in place. Within seconds, however, I broke into a run. What was I thinking? I had just a handful of commercials before I had to stand on that stage in a swimsuit!

All of our clothes had been moved for this high-speed change. But when I reached for my shoes, they weren't there. "Oh no!" I said to one of the hostesses. "Someone forgot to bring my shoes!" People scattered, looking frantically, while my name was yelled from the stage wing. I had to get on deck immediately. The commercial had just ended and the hosts were introducing the swimsuit segment. I couldn't believe this was happening. Suddenly, someone—I don't even know who—was sliding shoes on my feet. We got one on properly when I heard, "And now our first phase of competition begins. Let's welcome our first contestant..." We got my foot into the second shoe, but there was no time to buckle it. Someone tucked the strap in and a stagehand pushed me out from behind the curtain. Smile. Concentrate. Keep that shoe on. Turn. Keep smiling. Don't fall. My heart was pounding so hard from the speed of this last transition that I could feel it in my ears. What a start! Later, people commented that they had rarely seen a contestant walk with such grace in this phase of the competition. I guess the secret is being afraid your shoe will fall off and swinging your hips in a desperate effort to keep your feet steady. Who knew that grace and calamity went so well together!

After the swimsuit competition came the talent segment. Again, I was first. I got dressed with the help of the hostesses backstage, tested my blood sugar (all the while praying that it would remain stable throughout the competition), and started warming up my voice. This time, I made it to the stage with a few moments to spare. "This is it," I thought, "that second chance I asked for!" They called my name and I made my way to the middle of the stage. I stood with my back to the audience while my "Up Close and Personal" video played on the massive screen behind me. This video was shot right after I was named Miss Virginia. But this was the first time I had seen the tape. As I watched, I began to relax. I had been so rushed since they named the finalists that I had been focused on the competition. Now as I watched myself in segments of the video talking about my diabetes and my insulin pump, I remembered my mission. I was here to launch a platform—with this clip alone, my mission was already being accomplished.

As the video ended, I turned around to face the audience and sang "That's Life." I chose that song because it mirrored my struggle not to let obstacles or roadblocks stand in the way of accomplishments. After seeing that video, the audience would understand why I chose that song. This time, when I sang, I knew the message was getting through. I walked off the stage and felt that the performance had really come together.

Now came the easy part, the evening wear competition. All I had to do was walk, turn, and leave the stage. I did it and didn't trip. Victory!

After a commercial break, it was time to announce the next cut down to the top five. We stood together. Hearts pounding. I could hear mine. I almost believe I could hear all of our hearts. No one seemed to breathe. Miss Florida...Miss North Carolina...Miss Kentucky...Miss Missouri. With each passing place, I felt, *literally felt*, my chances shrinking, until, with the announcement of Miss Missouri, I did the unthinkable. I gave up. The tears welled up in my eyes. I was so close. My dream wouldn't become a reality. I braced myself for the next name that would personify my disappointment.

"Finally, the last semifinalist, Miss Virginia!" I jumped up and down, clapping my hands and trying to convince myself it was real! My head was spinning again—but I wasn't sick, it was just excitement—as I joined the line with the other four contestants.

Within seconds, the stage was transformed into a living room set for the final interview. Meredith Vieira, one of the cohosts of the talk show *The View*, would conduct it. She was a woman that I admired so much—a journalist of real depth and integrity. This time, I would be last. As we got started, the girls seemed nervous but still eloquent. But the questions were about living on a farm or what would you do if you were Hillary Clinton and your husband was named in headlines as having an affair. I thought these questions were not the right approach. I thought we should be asked about who we were and what we stood for. I didn't care what I was asked. I was going to talk about diabetes. As it turned out, I got my wish.

First, Meredith asked me what woman I admired most and why. Easy: "Elizabeth Dole, because although she is a woman with a high profile in politics, she is truly a woman of integrity. I admire her commitment to her husband and to her marriage." Then Meredith asked me about my diabetes. I smiled and felt relieved. As I talked about the disease I could sense that I was drawing the audience in. Everyone seemed incredibly quiet. I made a confession: "The biggest mistake I have ever made was being angry at God and turning my back on Him when I was diagnosed with diabetes.... I have come full circle and am now in great control, but it was very difficult at first." I thought that needed to be said to show that the struggle against diabetes was real and that it was hard.

After the final question, we were ushered off stage to change into our evening gowns once again. It was all over. I checked my blood sugar because adrenaline can significantly affect a person's glucose. My blood sugar was a little elevated so I pushed a button on my pump to give myself a little extra insulin. Then it was back to the task at hand and we lined up on stage. We were introduced one last time...and then cut to a commercial! I remember the audience sighing. I let out a breath of air I hadn't realized I was holding. We would all have to wait a few more minutes. Standing there, waiting, I heard, "Hey Virginia!" It was one of the judges. "Hey! Yeah you, Virginia!"

"Oh no. Oh no, what's happened now?" I thought.

It was Picabo Street, the downhill skier. I thought, "I'm not wearing the wrong shoes, am I?" But I nodded to her and quietly murmured, "Um, yes?"

She said, "So, are you wearing that pump right now?"

I thought I would die. Of course I was wearing the pump. I would have been in serious trouble if I hadn't been, with all of the adrenaline that was rushing through my body. I looked at her hesitantly and again nodded. She elbowed the judge next to her, Ian Ziering, one of the *Beverly Hills 90210* cast members, and said, "No way!" They were both looking at me now, and so was everyone else. Their next question was, "Well, where is it?" If I died of embarrassment from the first question, I died a second time now. I looked at them, smiled, and thought about it for a second, all the while trying to remain composed on that gigantic stage. I moved my hand slightly to motion to my thigh, saying through my teeth, "Right here."

They looked at me wide-eyed and started whispering to all the people around them. A few seconds later I heard, "Ten seconds to camera." We were back on the air.

The place started to vibrate, and it felt as if the roof would come right off. People were screaming. It was time to find out who would be the new Miss America.

The countdown began. "Fourth runner-up...Miss Kentucky....Third runner-up...Miss Missouri....Second runner-up, Miss Florida!"

I had always wondered what this would feel like. I looked at Miss North Carolina. We congratulated each other, but I couldn't feel anything. I was numb with excitement, yet there was also an uncanny peace in my spirit. At last we would know. I felt my muscles bracing. This was finally it.

Chapter 7

FULFILLING THE DREAM

"The first runner-up and winner of a $30,000 scholarship is Miss Nor..." That was all I heard. I jumped a foot off the ground. I raised my hands and thanked my Lord—the One I felt had brought me this far. Out of the corner of my eye I saw Kate Shindle, Miss America 1998, come over to me with the crown. I searched in vain for my family and state delegation in the audience. Eyes wide, head shaking, smile beaming, heart thumping, legs quivering, mind reeling. I thought the crown would never get on my head. When it was finally pinned and the scepter was handed to me, I lifted the hem of my dress slightly and stepped onto the runway—the first steps of the rest of my life.

That night was defining. It was life changing. It was monumental. It was everything I had always imagined it would be and so much more. I became Miss America, but more important, for the first time since being diagnosed with diabetes, I was comfortable with myself. I had proved that I could still achieve success. Even before being diagnosed I was always trying to improve myself: exercise, training, music and dance lessons, advancing my education. But now—now with the crown on my head—with the fulfillment of everything I had worked and hoped for, I felt not only wonderfully excited and happy, I finally felt content and confident. I was confident in my imperfection. And in that instant, I suddenly became a role model not only for millions of people with diabetes, but also for anyone with a chronic illness.

I knew that I was not a hero. My strength came from God, as did my simple good fortune. I know I am just a girl blessed with good genes. Ironically, of course, it was those very genes that also gave me a chronic medical condition. Diabetes very nearly claimed my life—until I learned to make it my life's purpose.

WHAT IT'S LIKE

When I got to the end of the runway, I finally spotted my family in the audience. I made eye contact, blew them a kiss, and then pirouetted into a whirlwind, which is the best word to describe my Miss America experience. I pledged to myself that the next 365 days would not be about me; they would be about the more than sixteen million Americans living with diabetes.

As I wiped away tears of joy, down came my fellow contestants—by now most were friends, even sisters—to congratulate me. I was hugged first by Miss New York, Deanna Herera (Deanna also has diabetes—we were both victorious that night). I wanted to savor the moment. Instead, the whirlwind, which would now dominate my life, blew me away.

Before I could even get to my other dear friends, two men grabbed my arms. For a brief moment a camera was in front of my face. Then I was propelled to another room where the national media were waiting for me to give the first live press conference in the history of the Miss America pageant.

I never understood why the press wanted to be in another room instead of capturing that moment on stage, where the whole auditorium could hear and enjoy it—or perhaps that *was* the reason; it made them feel exclusive. But because of the location, my family and friends missed the press conference. ABC broadcast it for only a few minutes, which was disappointing, because I used the press conference to talk about my passion and plans as they related to diabetes awareness.

After the press conference, I was escorted to another room backstage. I realized that I was surrounded by police escorts, security, and pageant officials. I was also followed by a Miss America Organization hostess and by my Virginia companion, Margaret. Together, Margaret, the Miss America staff, and the security people formed an impenetrable box around me. I guess I had an entourage for the first time.

We boarded a golf cart and rode through the halls of the convention center (thank God—my feet were killing me). Within moments, we arrived at a very cold room in the building's bowels. There was one chair, a small mirror, a compact, a hairbrush, some bobby pins, a diet drink, and somehow my meter was there. So I sat down to check my sugar, someone adjusted my crown, and then my family walked in. This was the first time I had seen them up close since winning. I told my mother she looked beautiful (she did). We could hardly contain our excitement, but we only had moments together before I was taken from this unglamorous dressing room into a bewildering maze of elevators and unfamiliar hallways. We came out of the maze just outside a visitation room, and I instinctively reached for the doorknob. A hand reached out to stop me, and I was held outside the "visitation hall" by security, while they swept the room before I entered. Then they announced me by my title as I was led forward amid deafening applause and cheers to speak briefly to the other contestants, their families, and members of the various state delegations. I saw flash bulbs snapping pictures and heard shouts of "Miss America, Miss America, congratulations!" Despite the security, many people had pushed their way not only to the front of the room but onto the stage. What a feeling—and not necessarily a good one. I was bewildered by the commotion. I was still the same person who had just minutes before been one of a million girls who dreamed of one day being Miss America. Now, suddenly, I felt quite different, part of me kept thinking that I belonged in the crowd with everyone else. I have no idea what I said, but when I concluded there was blaring music, the Miss America song, being played for me! My entourage bustled me away again. I felt I was trapped in a flood, swept along, helpless. BUT WAIT! *I want to see my state delegation, my friends, my family.* I soon learned that what I wanted—even in this moment of triumph—didn't matter; I was Miss America, with a job to do and scheduled obligations to fulfill.

Next stop was the ABC party with all the bigwigs—ABC executives, important guests, and former Miss Americas. Everyone stopped and clapped and cheered as I walked in. I was asked to sign autographs and have photos taken (all firsts for me as Miss America 1999), but I was so tired—and where was my family? I just wanted to sit down, but I couldn't. I was now public property, with an all-important image to maintain.

I was the closest thing there is to American royalty—complete with crown—and the unreported truth about royalty, though I could have read it in any book on the subject, is that your time is never your own. With the crown comes responsibility. Actually, one of the best preparations for being Miss America, though I didn't know it at the time, would be to read the history plays of Shakespeare.

Anyway, after a short extemporaneous speech to the guests at the party and a slew of photos, I was led to Harrah's, my host hotel, where yet another crowd was waiting for me. To be honest, I'm still not sure who these people were, though some of my family members—aunts and uncles—made it there. They tried to congratulate me but were again stopped by security. Untouched by family, unable to talk to whom I wanted, forbidden to greet friends and supporters—I was like a fairy princess, surrounded by an impenetrable shield of armed knights, about to be locked into a tower.

If you are ever going to be locked in a tower, this was the one to be in. To say it was a pleasant tower would be a major understatement. I was taken inside to a high-roller suite with food, champagne, sodas, and, of course, more security. I'd never been in such a luxurious place. I couldn't believe there was a hot tub right smack in the middle of the living room and a tanning bed in one of the three bathrooms! I couldn't believe that it had THREE bathrooms. My parents arrived and eventually convinced the security guards to allow my extended family into the room—my mother's six brothers and sisters with their spouses and some of my cousins. For the first time that night I was with people who were not pulling at me or taking pictures of me. I was finally with the people who really knew me and could share my joy. For the first time I was able to cry, scream, jump, yell, and cheer with abandon. We posed for family photos, enjoyed a toast, and mingled until about 2:30 A.M. The room cleared out and I thought about soaking in the hot tub and maybe even catching some rays in the tanning bed, but I knew time was short. I had only three hours before I needed to be up for the traditional morning-after, romp-on-the-beach photographs. So I settled for a very quick, very hot shower. When I came out of the shower, I was surprised to find three ladies waiting for me. One was Margaret. I thought the other two were just lingerers from the party, but when I was about to ask them to leave, Margaret advised me that they were armed. They were my bodyguards. More security! I also learned there was a security guard packing heat outside the door. They actually slept in my room that night—to make sure nothing happened to the new Miss America. Because Atlantic City is full of so many people during pageant week, that first night and the following morning is always a sensitive time. The next morning they, with even more security, accompanied me to the beach.

BEGINNINGS

I woke up looking at my crown. It was on the pillow beside me, and I thought, "You mean, I wasn't dreaming?" I lay there with a satisfied grin on my face. This was real. I really was Miss America. Maybe just a few more minutes of sleep...

Margaret came into the room and said, "Time to wake up, Miss America."

Splashing around in the cold waters of the Atlantic Ocean at the crack of dawn will wake anyone. When I arrived at the beach, I was immediately surrounded by the usual—at least I'd learned it was usual—mobs of security, police, and other officials.

The press were already assembled on the beach for the official photo shoot—yelling reporters and flashing cameras—when I arrived. I wondered briefly if they had slept at all during the night. I almost felt like a panda in the zoo—a trained panda. They made me sit in the sand, run on the beach, and jump around like a happy-go-lucky all-American girl. I *was* sincerely excited about being Miss America, but even an all-American girl can feel a little less than lustrous at six o'clock in the morning on a cold, wet beach in New Jersey. Sometimes, though, you just can't break with tradition—nor do you want to.

After the photo shoot, I had about an hour to get back to my room, clean up (I had salt water and sand all over me), get dressed, and swallow some food before I was expected at my first meetings at the Miss America offices. I was especially looking forward to meeting with Leonard Horn, CEO of the Miss America Organization, who had just resigned. He had served for many years, and I had heard so many good stories about him. He was a wonderful person, and we had a delightful meeting, tinged with a little sadness because of his imminent departure.

On to other offices, other meetings. I was inundated with so many contracts, waivers, and other paperwork to sign that I literally didn't have time to read them myself, let alone have an attorney look at them. So, basically, I signed my life away to the organization for the next 365 days. But that really didn't bother me. This was what I had wanted, to be Miss America, and I was content—if hyperventilating a bit—to sign all the papers and jump through every hoop they set for me. I was still so excited, bright-eyed (the beach *had* helped wake me up), and thrilled to be beginning this new journey, that I probably would have signed absolutely anything.

Especially since I was a budding journalist, what I found more interesting than the paperwork was the sudden national media spotlight that fell on me. I had never really been on this side of the media before. The brief news conference after the pageant had been one thing. But I soon discovered that the media—and, apparently, the public—wanted my opinion on more than just diabetes and the Miss America Organization. I was suddenly, in public forums, asked for advice on how to raise children, run the country, and solve the world's crises. My past was investigated—again, in public. The tabloids camped out in my parents' neighborhood to get any morsel of information they could about my early years—they even stole yearbooks from my high school! Of course, there were no skeletons in my closet. The worst scandal the press could come up with was that I performed with a girls' choir that was badly dressed and had big hair!

As luck would have it, I was crowned Miss America during a time when the newspapers were filled with stories about scandals in the administration of President Bill Clinton. At my next national press conference, I certainly wasn't in as much hot water as he was, facing possible impeachment over the Monica Lewinsky affair and other issues, but I still felt the heat. When the press conference started, I made an opening statement about diabetes, my dedication to working for a cure, and my plans for the future. An AP reporter stood up and asked, "Nicole, we had a survey going around to all the contestants during the Miss America week asking whether they thought President Clinton should resign or should he be impeached or did they care not to comment." He pulled out a sheet of paper and said, "You, Nicole, declined to give an opinion or comment at that time. I want to know what your position is now because obviously Miss America has to have an opinion on this topic. What would you choose? Should the president resign or be impeached?"

Tricky. But I've never succumbed to pressures of political correctness, and I certainly didn't want to show that type of weakness now, as Miss America. I always thought it best to be honest and not to sugarcoat or cover up what I thought was the truth, so I answered that I felt it would be better for the president to resign rather than be impeached. President Clinton's actions, I said, were shameful, and it was sad that an individual in a position as a role model, particularly for children, would compromise his responsibility like that.

Needless to say, I wasn't invited to the White House as is customary for Miss America. I quickly learned that this ride was going to be a bumpy one.

After that press conference, I waved to my parents across the lobby. I was hoping to see them for lunch later, but as it turned out I wouldn't see them again for several weeks. I went back to Harrah's to find my suitcases and belongings were gone! Margaret told me I had half an hour to order something from room service before I left for New York City to meet other officials from the Miss America Organization! Then she kissed me, said she was proud of me, told me I'd be getting a new traveling companion, and waved goodbye. The whirlwind suddenly became very still and quiet.

I ordered some oatmeal and ate it alone in my room. The continual changes were difficult to adjust to. But the Miss America Organization had new traveling companions already picked out—two women who would switch off every month and who would become my two new "best" friends for the next year.

EARLY TURBULENCE

I climbed into the limo and got to know Bonnie, one of my new traveling companions. She was a pretty redhead who frequently reminded me that I was the tenth Miss America she had handled. She tended to be very protective—more protective than I was used to. She told me I could fall asleep on the ride to New York because that's what all the other Miss Americas did. I didn't need convincing—I was exhausted. Of course, once I dozed off, Bonnie took the customary photo of Miss America, with a newspaper gently lying across her chest or backside, dozing.

The legendary Miss America suite at the Intercontinental Hotel in New York was under construction, so I didn't get to stay there. But the alternative suite the hotel provided was heavenly. It was decorated Victorian-style in pinks, greens, and blues—the same way my house was decorated in my daydreams (with a wonderful husband and beautiful children, of course). While I felt as if I was adapting to these new surroundings, I also had a sense of anxiety: everything was so surprising and new, and I felt so alone and unsure of myself. I wanted to do a good job. I wanted to make a good impression. I wanted to prove myself worthy of being there.

"I can't believe you started off your year this way! I can't believe your comments about the president of the United States! Do you know what people are saying about you? They're saying Miss America is part of a vast right-wing conspiracy!" So much for making a good impression and proving myself worthy. The barrage of verbal insults were coming from none other than the organization's "media trainer." My insides churned as he continued the browbeating. I started to cry. Then he told me I needed to change my position on politics—

actually, to be nonpolitical and nonpartisan—throughout my year as Miss America, and he told me I needed speech training.

The tears stopped. I lifted my chin. I wasn't nervous anymore. I was indignant. I was happy to represent the Miss America Organization to the best of my ability, and I understood the need to be diplomatic, but I wouldn't ever fudge the truth. I would give straight answers to straight and unavoidable questions. I wouldn't be told what to believe. I didn't say this out loud, but I was thinking it. I realized that while we can all use improvement in every area of our lives, I knew I didn't need full-blown speech training. I'd been a successful public speaker all of my adult life. I had a master's degree in journalism. I had already traveled extensively representing the issue of diabetes. While I did need some guidance to help me deal with the special problems associated with being Miss America, I didn't need a lot of handholding or media training to be effective. I knew the talent of my speaking lay in the spontaneity, honesty, and heartfelt nature of my words—not in the planning and preprogramming of a media trainer, especially one with this much tact and finesse. His method of dealing with me had offended me greatly, and I knew that training with him would not be fruitful. I did suck it up and give it the old college try, but my instincts were right, and it was basically a waste of time.

I also understood that Miss America represented all people, but I didn't think the country, or the organization for that matter, wanted a Miss America who would change her views, feelings, morals, and values so easily. I was going to be Nicole Johnson, someone with a strong moral character and someone who knew what she stood for and wasn't afraid to say it. In addition, I knew exactly where I would be as Miss America if

I ever behaved as immorally as President Clinton. There would be no Senate hearings, no impeachment debates. I would be quickly and severely removed from my role—and rightly so. Tact I was willing to learn, but I would never fudge what I believed to be the truth.

As I left the "media training," I felt rejected. I went to my room to get dressed for dinner and broke down in sobs. I called my family and told them I didn't want to be Miss America. My dreams had shattered. What I had hoped would be the fulfillment of all the work, competitions, and training—everything I'd done to make myself a better person, everything I'd done so that I could help others—had suddenly been reduced from dreamlike splendor to a nightmare of struggle. I wasn't competing anymore. I was done with the criticisms. This was supposed to be fun. This was supposed to be serious work where lives would be improved and even saved. My parents, of course, were voices of reason and patience; they listened while I blew out my frustrations. In the end, they and my faith helped me recover.

The Miss America Organization was in charge. They decided which events I would attend and which events I would not. They decided how long I would stay at those events. The organization decided if, and for how long, I could let individuals take photos of me or let me sign autographs. In essence, they determined whom I could talk to at a public event. To me, not having been under such public scrutiny before, the "control" aspect, at times, seemed ridiculous. I was shocked to find that often I wasn't even allowed to decide what I was going to wear. When I did get to choose, I could count on criticism for my choice of dress or hairstyle.

It is unfortunate, but true, that a day didn't go by as Miss America that I didn't feel like a caged bird. Just a few days into my reign I was taken to the hairdresser. I had always dreamed of getting my hair cut by a New York stylist. I thought this was the height of glamour—definitely one of the perks of my new position. But they sat me in a chair, with no mirror in front of me, and proceeded to cut away. What I was led to believe was going to be a "trim" of my fairly long hair turned out to be a whole new hairdo: short hair with short bangs. I had as much say in the matter as if I'd been a pet poodle. Here I am, the new Miss America, with a "new look" I didn't even ask for. What was wrong with my old look? I won Miss America with my old look! Everyone tried to tell me that my new hairdo looked good, but it didn't. It was embarrassing. Eventually, I found ways to make the best of my new, shorter hairstyle. I remained very positive publicly about the new and improved Nicole, but by the end of the year I was glad that my hair was long again.

So there I was: trained in communications, being told I needed speech training; having won with beautiful long hair, now sporting some fancy short do. Now I stared in disbelief as Miss America Organization representatives stood in my hotel suite telling me to scrap the diabetes issue. "Maybe you should think about changing your platform, Nicole. We just don't know what we can do with it, how we can make it work, and how we can market it. I don't think this is going to be possible."

I thought: "This is it! This is unbelievable! This is not going to happen! The only reason I wanted to become Miss America was *because* of my platform!" I was in the midst of a battle. I stood up straight, looked them in the eye, and told them changing the platform was not an option. Luckily, I was able to convince them that we could make it work.

I know that part of the problem was that many of the people in the organization didn't understand diabetes. They were afraid of it—and they were treating me very differently because of it. They had never had to deal with a Miss America who had a disease, and they were treating me as if I were sick. I believe that they were genuinely concerned about me and wanted to protect me—I love them for that—and they were also concerned about the image of Miss America. It took several months before people started to relax and see that I was in control of my condition. In fact, one of my traveling companions wrote a letter to my family confessing that she had worried too much about my having diabetes but had eventually learned that I knew how to take care of myself—in her words, I was "the master."

One of my trademarks while serving as Miss America was a gold medallion bracelet. One side has the caduceus, the international medical symbol of two entwined serpents that comes from Greek mythology. The other side says "Type I Diabetic." It is my medical identification to make sure that emergency medical technicians and paramedics know how to take care of me in case of an emergency. I was and am proud to wear the bracelet, and I'm a big advocate of wearing medical IDs in general. That medallion—and even more important, simple experience—helped me put the fears of the Miss America Organization and my traveling companions to rest. It took a little while, however, for me to chase my own fears away and to trust that all these Miss America Organization handlers and advisers wanted me to succeed just as much as I did.

LOWLIGHTS

As experienced as I was in controlling my diabetes, I did, however, have one hospital experience as Miss America. My hospital trip was not diabetes related, but I didn't know that at the time. It was during the spring of 1999 and I was running

from event to event like crazy. I was on a marathon of appearances. One day, I was in a hotel somewhere in Connecticut,
and after working through the morning, I started feeling odd.
I ordered lunch thinking some nourishment might be the
remedy, but when it arrived I had no appetite. The smell of
the food actually made my stomach curl. I figured I was just
fatigued, and maybe I simply needed to relax a little. I called
the gym, got a referral for a massage, and had the hotel van
take me to the massage studio to treat myself.

Well, while I was there the pain in my stomach got worse.
I couldn't bear to be touched in my abdomen—it felt like it
was going to explode (so much for my massage). I returned to
the hotel and quickly fell asleep. I was so tired and worn out.
But who wouldn't be with only one day off a month? As the
night wore on, my blood sugar rose, which wasn't new—I had
been having high blood sugar readings as a result of the travel,
inconsistent schedule, and stress which all come with the territory for any Miss America. Then I started vomiting and
quickly became dehydrated. Bonnie, ever cautious about my
condition, decided to call for an ambulance. I resisted for fear
someone would recognize me or make a big deal about the
fact that I was sick. But thinking back on previous diabetic
episodes, I started to get a little worried. Virtually every time
I had had problems, they began with similar symptoms. So I
finally consented (in the event, she thought better of it and
had a hotel van take us). Since I didn't want my diabetes to
become a public spectacle, I asked Bonnie not to tell anyone
who I was. I didn't want a press leak, like the one during my
time as Miss Virginia, when I had the flu and somehow word
spread that I was at the hospital, causing a bit of a scene. But
Bonnie had already called ahead and told the hospital that

Miss America was coming in with a medical emergency. I did get a private room in the hospital and had a few doctors assist me—it was obviously special treatment—but I was horrified. I guess I had a little too much pride, something I struggle with on a daily basis. While I tell myself that I don't want to be a bother, sometimes it's pride that keeps me from accepting help.

Luckily, this time my illness wasn't some complication from the diabetes. According to the doctors, all that I had was a virus complicated by the fact that my body was malnourished and in a state of exhaustion. Ugh. I was in the hospital for only one night; I was relieved that it wasn't anything more serious. I still hoped to keep a low profile and not let word leak out that Miss America had been hospitalized. But Bonnie was one step ahead of me again, knowing that I couldn't stay anonymous. She had pulled out autograph cards and had me sign photos for the hospital staff and doctors before I left.

That whole night in the hospital, Bonnie and I were on the phone with the Miss America Organization. Together with the organization, we decided that I should go back to the hotel and carry on with the schedule I had for the next morning. They told me the events took planning and money and to cancel suddenly would be a "disaster," so I flew from Connecticut to California and then on to Arizona in the next two days. A cross-country flight was probably the last thing I should have done, but it exemplifies the philosophy: Miss America is *not* allowed to get sick. There just isn't time. I managed to give three speeches in California the next day, but our clients there didn't understand the necessity of giving me more rest than originally scheduled. With the best intentions, they wanted me to mingle and to have the opportunity to chat; they thought that just allowing me to sit in a quiet room in between speeches was enough. It wasn't—and it took a lot longer to recover from the virus than I thought it would. But then, again, I had lots of surprises as Miss America.

Chapter 8

HIGHLIGHTS

The Miss America journey wasn't without conflict or difficulties, and while these make good reading with all of their drama and surprise, it is far from the whole story. My time as Miss America was full of great (sometimes crazy) moments, and I met some wonderful people along the way. One special moment was on the set of *Good Morning America*, the Monday after I'd won the title. I wasn't interviewed by Charlie Gibson or Diane Sawyer—a woman whose career and broadcast presence I admire greatly—but by Lisa McRee and Kevin Newman. Knowing my background in broadcast journalism, they let me read from the teleprompter as a temporary anchorwoman. That was a kind gesture on their part and fun to do.

After the *Good Morning America* interview, I went to one of the other ABC studios and taped a show for *The View*. It was there that I met Barbara Walters, Star Jones, Debbie

Matenopoulos, and Joy Behar. Meredith Vieira was also there. I was a bit intimidated because these women can be tough interviewers; we've all seen them reduce people virtually to tears. But they were wonderfully kind to me. Of course, they did ask about my comments regarding President Clinton (every media program and every interview over the next two months brought that up). Ironically, the videotapes of President Clinton's testimony on the Monica Lewinsky affair were released the same day my spot on *The View* was supposed to appear. So I was bumped by President Clinton. I guess he got back at me.

It was only my third day as Miss America when I found myself a guest on *The Tonight Show* and the brunt of a big joke Jay Leno played on me about my President Clinton comments. A Clinton look-alike was waiting for me outside when I arrived. I thought I would have a heart attack! Was I ever going to live this down? Sometimes you just have to laugh at yourself... even on a very public stage.

Another cool, fun, glamorous moment of being Miss America was visiting New York designers for the complimentary Miss America wardrobe. Granted, they weren't the kind of clothes I would normally buy for myself, but I was thankful nonetheless. I didn't come from an affluent background, and I didn't have a vast wardrobe when I became Miss America. I had been a struggling student. But now I received beautiful suits from Kaspar, who traditionally gives Miss America the outfits she wears during her speaking tours, five or six things from ChetaB, and three outfits from Alberto Makali. Among the gifts were several fabulous winter coats. (My favorite Miss America gift, however, was a leather portfolio to carry my speeches in. I still use it for meetings and speaking engagements.)

I wanted to wear all the new clothes while on the road, but unfortunately, as Miss America you are only allowed to travel with two suitcases. Whatever I could fit in those suitcases I took with me; everything else was shipped home. Occasionally, I would FedEx something home in exchange for a suit I wanted. Although I was already used to packing for trips of four or five days at a time, being on the road constantly presented other problems. What do you do about laundry if you're traveling practically 365 days a year? I found out that, when you're Miss America, you don't get to go home to wash your clothes, and you don't really have access to a washing machine or a dryer. Believe it or not, in my first week as Miss America one of my biggest duties was to find some Woolite to carry in one of my two allotted suitcases. If you peered into my hotel room most nights you would have found Miss America on her hands and knees in the bathroom, bubbles flying everywhere, washing out my necessities, clothes, and pantyhose in the bathtub with my trusty Woolite. Sometimes in desperation, if I had run out of Woolite, I'd use shampoo. That's ingenuity for you.

You may be wondering, why didn't I just send my clothes out to be cleaned. Well, I was changing locations every twenty-four to thirty-six hours. Sometimes I was in a city for less than twenty-four hours. Usually, there wasn't enough time to send anything out or have it dry-cleaned by the hotel. That presented another problem. My mom and I quickly solved that problem by developing an ingenious system where I would FedEx her my dirty clothes in exchange for clean ones. Whenever I FedExed something home, I'd have to have my mom replace it with something similar because I never knew what kind of events I'd be going to next. Mom and I would have to coordinate so that our packages—containing dresses or underwear or workout T-shirts—arrived simultaneously.

I wound up separating my things in terms of travel. In one suitcase I packed four business suits, a couple of pantsuits, an evening gown (or a cocktail dress), shoes to go with the suits, a winter coat (in case we went to a cold climate), clothes suitable for warmer weather, and formal athletic gear for walkathons. The other suitcase carried my tennis shoes, medical supplies, Woolite, a couple of books, casual travel clothing, and some bum-around workout gear. It was a very interesting balancing act. My traveling companions also had two suitcases each (and between us, we took all the carry-ons we could get away with). That's why one of the requirements of Miss America is that she be picked up or chauffeured in a limo—not because we're pretentious divas, but because we have to transport all that darn luggage.

That luggage was not only a pain to lug around, it became the source of a long-running bad joke. Many people made fun, on a daily basis, of the weight and size of the suitcases. I know it sounds trivial, but every single time I would land in an airport the skycap or somebody else would say, "Oh, this suitcase must be for all your shoes," or "Is this one for all your makeup?" It was funny at first, but hearing the same lines day in and day out drove me crazy. (The suitcases weighed about seventy pounds each, so you can imagine why the skycaps hated us.)

One of my worst experiences as Miss America was when I found myself standing on a baggage belt trying to rearrange the contents of my suitcases to the satisfaction of an overzealous ticket agent. Admittedly, one of my two Tumi suitcases was overweight by three pounds—but the other suitcase was underweight by four pounds! So, I had to rearrange my luggage until each bag weighed exactly what it should. Usually, when my luggage was a little overweight, we would slip the agent an autographed photo and things would be overlooked. I was never more than about five pounds over the weight limit, even though I was constantly given books, T-shirts, mugs, and other gifts on the road. Every other week, I would send home a box full of goodies.

I found out the hard way that sometimes even Miss America is subject to travel nightmares. I have been stranded in countless airports throughout the country. One night I found myself stuck in Atlanta. After waiting for hours, our flight to Tennessee was cancelled, and Bonnie and I had to hire a car—at 2 A.M.—to drive us to our next location. We couldn't wait for a flight the next day since I was scheduled to give a speech in Tennessee at 10 A.M.! Well, we arrived around 5 A.M. and there was just enough time for a short nap before the event. Fortunately, while I was waiting in the airport before the flight was cancelled, I had had the forethought to spend the time sitting on the baggage belt with my laptop and typing out my speech for the next morning. I've slept in many airports around the country—once next to the baggage belt, once on chairs, once right on the floor at the terminal. You name it, I've slept there.

I've also had my share of crazy limo experiences. At one appearance during my year as Miss America, Bonnie and I were in a limo going from the airport to the hotel, and our driver started going down the wrong side of the highway! I didn't scream—I guess I was too stunned—but I grabbed Bonnie's hand and started praying. My other hand was holding on for dear life. Thank goodness it was late and there weren't many cars on the road. And then there was the time I had to give a speech to a large group of physicians at the Diabetes Treatment Centers of America conference in Key Largo, Florida. We were in the midst of a tropical storm and as we were checking into the hotel, the power suddenly went out, leaving us in complete darkness. After several hours, we found a flashlight, climbed the stairs to our room, and then proceeded to feast on the snacks we found in the minibar for lack of any alternative. With no power for hours, I finally decided to hang it up and go to bed when I lost the battery power of my computer and cell phone.

The ultimate limo experience, however, was a white and red velvet limo in Sioux City, Iowa, driven by this Harley guy who must have told all his Harley friends that he was driving Miss America around. I had to make several stops throughout the city, and every time I stepped out of the car the same rough-looking dudes and dudettes were outside waiting for me. At first, they were just standing there staring at me. But after several stops they started taking pictures of me in what I felt were compromising positions (getting out of the car, bending over—you know what I mean). I know they were having a lot of fun, but when I began to feel uncomfortable, my companion asked if they would lay off—which they kindly did.

BARE NECESSITIES

There was an additional complication to what is, under any circumstances, a hectic life. As I traveled, I had to keep a constant supply of diabetes medical supplies coming my way. This meant that about a quarter of my luggage space was taken up with medical supplies. These supplies were FedExed to me by Minimed—the manufacturer of my insulin pump. Because I was traveling all the time, I wasn't able to go to my doctor or my regular pharmacy to have prescriptions refilled, or to get pump supplies. I would send Minimed a list of three hotels where I was going to be for the next four or five days, and they would calculate how long the supplies would take to get to me, timing the shipment so that the supplies would be waiting for me at my destination. The people at Minimed were my angels! They would also send medical supplies to the Miss America office in Atlantic City, so when my traveling companions (Bonnie and Mickey) switched off, which was on a monthly basis, they would bring me additional supplies. It really took a lot of planning. I got to know the different rules and regulations of the insurance industry very well. My doctor and I had to become even better acquainted, as I often had to lean on him for assistance during my travels around the country. Many times I would be standing in a pharmacy in some place like Foley, Alabama, handing my cell phone to the pharmacist so my doctor could tell the pharmacist directly to fill my prescriptions. That's how I would get my insulin while I was on the road. Occasionally, pharmacists gave us some problems, but most of the time it worked. When it comes to your personal health, sometimes you need to be a little feisty to get what you need. That and having access to your medical team is essential.

PRIVACY IS A THING OF THE PAST
But even having the peace of mind of a reliable medical team changed when I became Miss America. In the past, when life got crazy or if I was under a lot of stress and I hit some turbulence in regulating my blood glucose, I could always depend on my next doctor's visit to set things straight. Sometimes my doctor would help adjust my insulin pump.

Other times he'd just give me a pep talk when I needed it. The doctor's office was my health sanctuary—a place where I could go to share my most private worries about my diabetes. But suddenly, when I became Miss America, I went from being just a private patient to a patient that people could talk about. Now, they weren't just taking care of me—Nicole—they were taking care of Miss America. I can't say I ever got used to this loss of privacy, but it was a fact.

In one instance I was in Pennsylvania and needed to have my A1C measured, the glucose average test that I have every three months. As I was waiting for the results, I noticed a crowd had gathered. Was there a medical discovery—maybe a cure of some kind? No such luck. Everyone was just eager to see what Miss America's A1C checked out to be.

I still struggle with going to see medical doctors or endocrinologists for fear that someone will share my private medical information with others. Part of the fear is that they will judge me on what my diabetes control is like or what my levels are during that particular visit. I had to battle against that fear constantly—and still do. I so wanted to be a good role model, but everyday circumstances—when your every move is watched—made me very conscious of how hard it can be to always appear perfect. I am just beginning to realize that this is not necessary, that being too concerned about how others regard you interferes with the trust and confidence necessary for true friendships to develop.

I found that even simple tasks, like purchasing curlers and feminine products, were no longer so simple. As I traveled, the simple act of shopping required getting sponsors to make those arrangements—and to accompany me to the store. As one who is intent on keeping her personal life personal, I

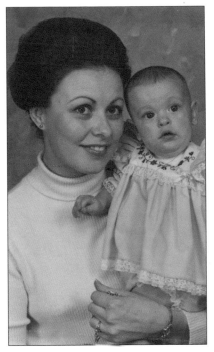

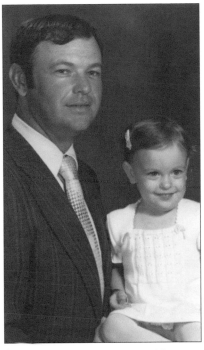

If only you knew how much of a handful I really was.

Daddy's little girl at two years old.

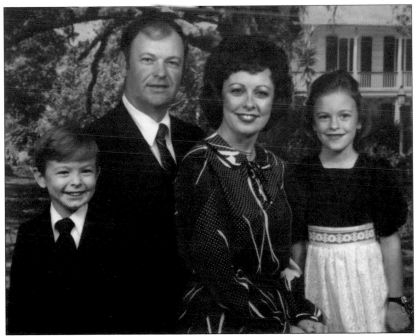

My sweet family.

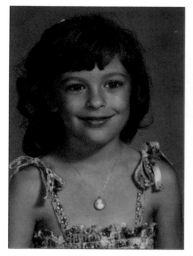

Kindergarten days.

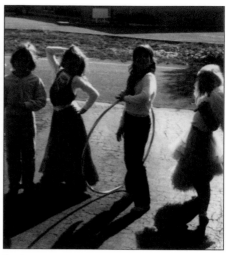

Perfecting "The Pose" during my eighth
birthday party.

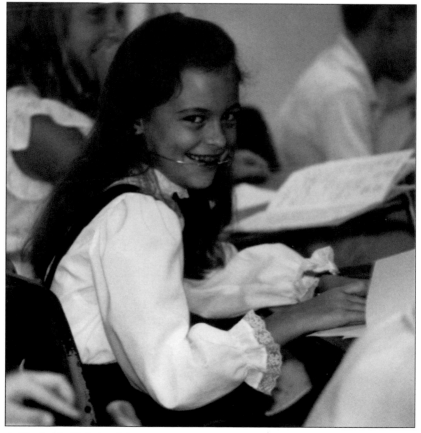

At Northside Christian School.

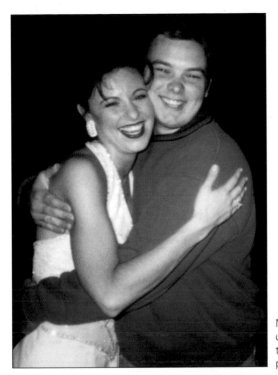

My precious brother, Scott, congratulating me on winning the Miss Apple Blossom pageant in 1997.

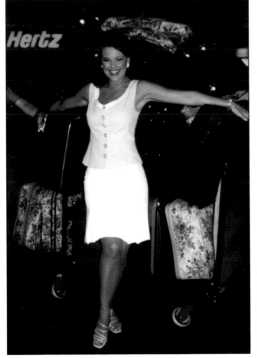

All packed and ready to go to the Miss America competition—three weeks' worth of luggage for me and my official traveling companion. As a touring Miss America, I'd be limited to two bags and two carry-ons.

The Miss America Evening Wear Competition.

Singing "That's Life" during the Talent Competition.

Thanking my Lord
for the opportunity
to serve as Miss America.

A dream come true.

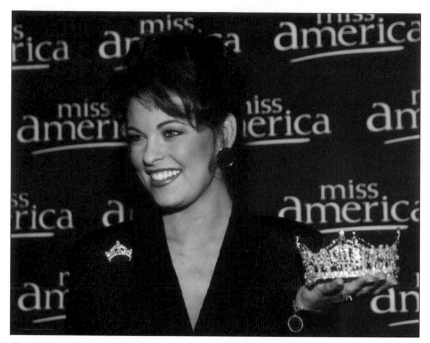

The national press conference the morning after the pageant.

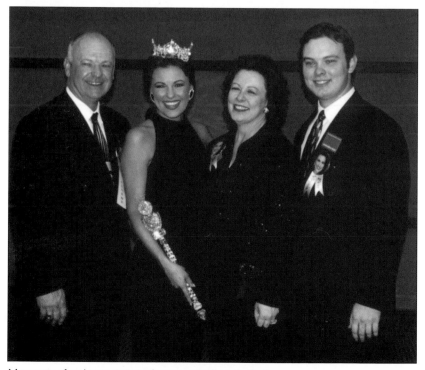

Moments after I was crowned: we were all so thrilled.

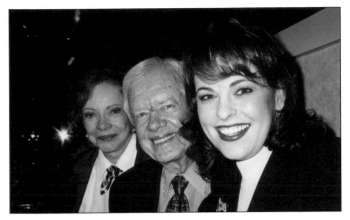

Spending time with former president Jimmy Carter and former first lady Rosalynn Carter at Super Bowl XXXIII.

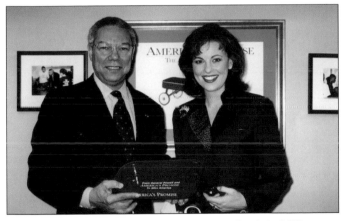

Promoting health care with General Colin Powell to help fulfill "America's Promise."

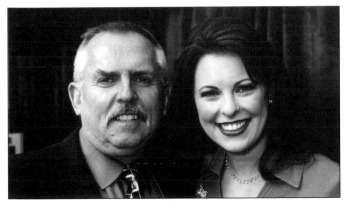

With John Ratzenberger, of *Cheers* fame, who touched my heart in a special way when he shared his son's struggle with diabetes.

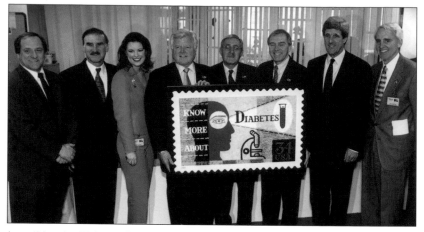

Launching the Diabetes Awareness Stamp in March 2001 at the
Joslin Diabetes Center in Boston.

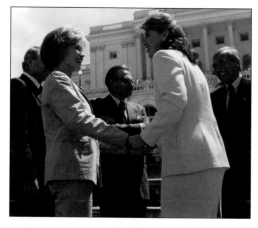

On the steps of the Capitol with
Mary Tyler Moore, Larry King,
and Congressman
George Nethercutt at the
JDRF's First Children's Congress
in 1999.

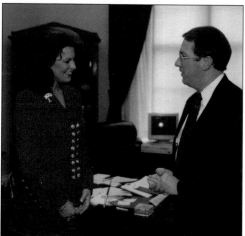

Lobbying for diabetes funding
with Congressman
Bob Goodlatte of Virginia.

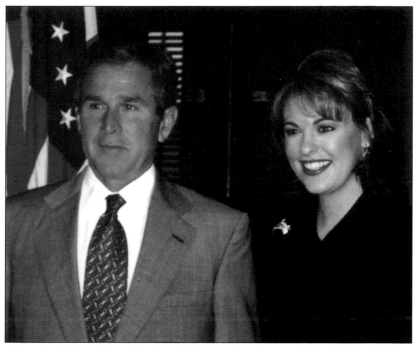

Discussing diabetes related issues with then-governor George W. Bush in Austin, Texas.

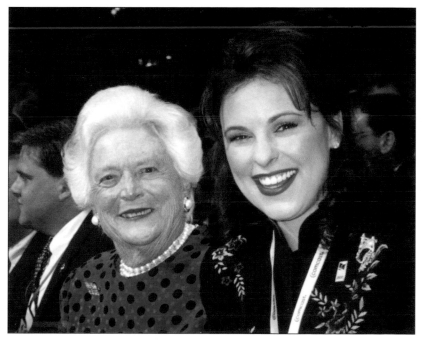

Sharing a memorable moment at the 2000 Republican National Convention with former first lady Barbara Bush.

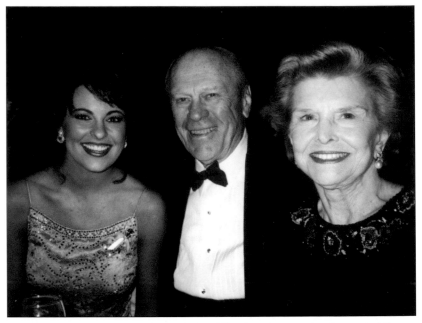

The most star-studded event I attended as Miss America was the Carousel of Hope Ball in Los Angeles. Here I am sharing dinner with former president Gerald Ford and former first lady Betty Ford.

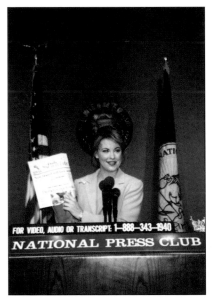

It was a great honor to be invited to speak at the National Press Club in an event that was broadcast nationally by C-SPAN, helping me get the word out about diabetes.

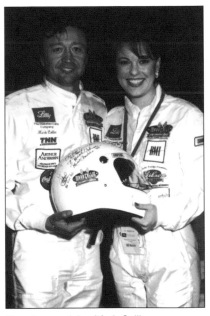

Country musician Mark Collie, my friend and fellow diabetic, at his annual diabetes fundraising race. (For more info see www.markcollie.org.)

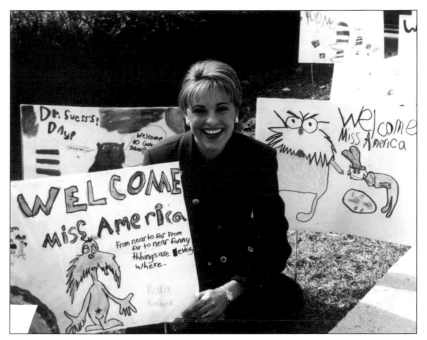

Diabetes wasn't my only cause. Promoting literacy was another.
Here I am in Chicago for *"Cat In the Hat* Day."

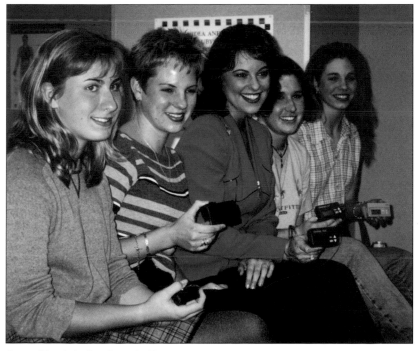

Pump friends in San Antonio, Texas.

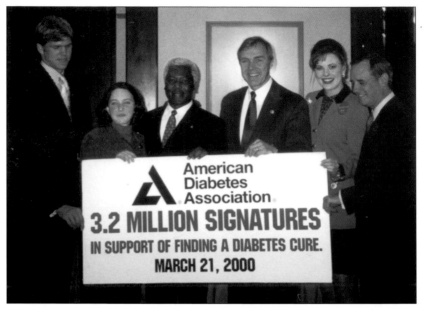

With Olympian Gary Hall, Jr., Clare Rosenfeld, Ed Hawthorne (past chairman of the American Diabetes Association), Congressman George Nethercutt, and John Graham

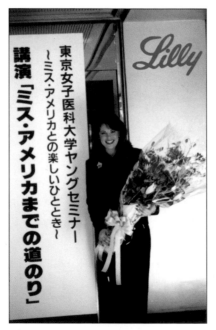

After my term as Miss America, Eli Lilly and Company sent me to fifteen countries, including Japan, to promote diabetes care and awareness.

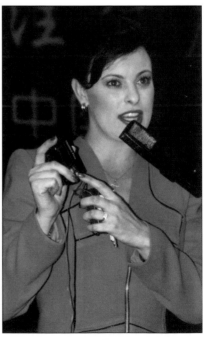

MiniMed, Inc., manufacturer of my insulin pump, sent me to China to educate people about the benefits of pump therapy.

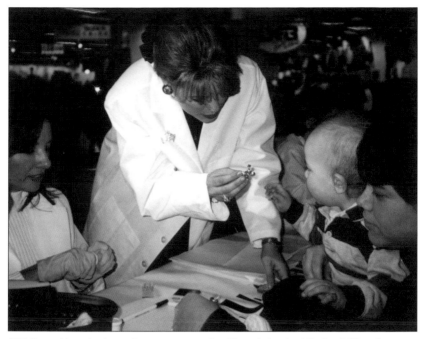

Eli Lilly and I worked together to promote the "Search for the Missing Millions" campaign, which offered free diabetes screenings in thirteen states across the country.

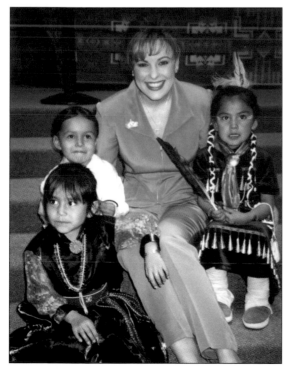

With some of my friends at the Navajo Nation. Native Americans have an especially high incidence of diabetes.

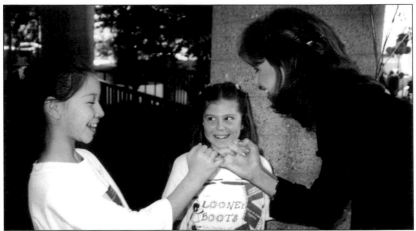

Sharing a pinky promise with a young friend with diabetes in Portland, Oregon. She's taking a pledge to stay healthy, check her glucose levels often, and never let the disease get her down.

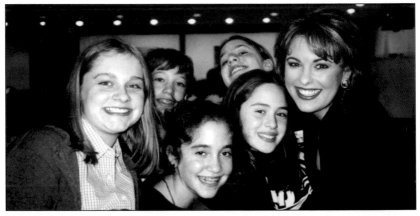

Making friends at the United Nations peace forum.

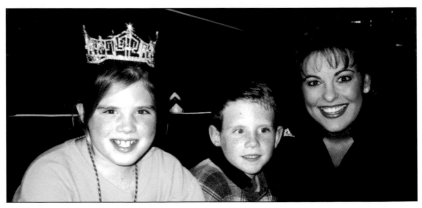

I invited some kids to go for a spin in the limo after an event in North Carolina.

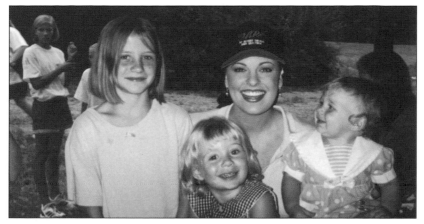

At a D.A.R.E. event in Roanoke, Virginia, in 1998.

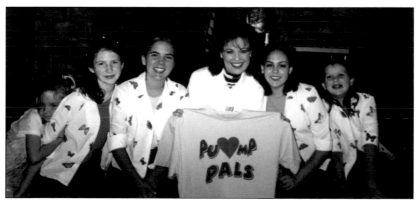

Promoting F.U.N. Fitness (Families Understanding Nutrition and Fitness) in Tampa, Florida.

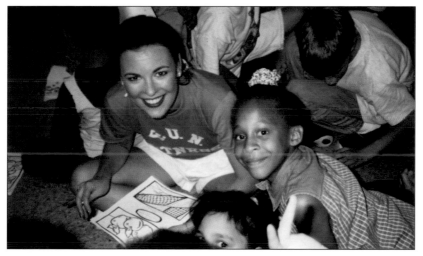

Jamming with the Pump Girls!

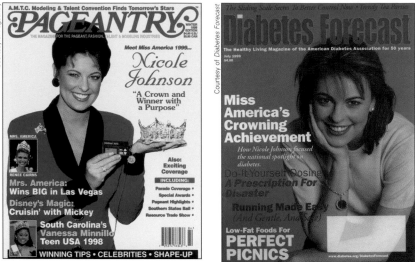

I was selected to be on the cover of *Pageantry* in December 1998 and *Diabetes Forecast* in June 1999.

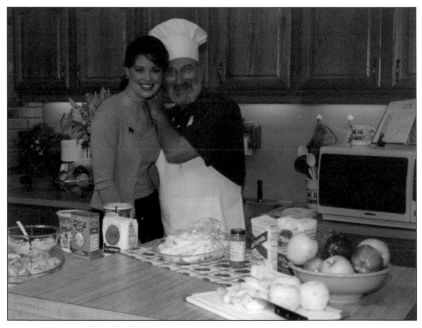

Cooking up a storm with my kitchen buddy, Mr. Food (Art Ginsburg), for our *Mr. Food's Quick & Easy Diabetic Cooking (Featuring Nicole Johnson): Over 150 Recipes Everybody Will Love.*

found it difficult to purchase private items under the watchful eyes of strangers. To give you another example of just how extreme the lack of privacy could be, I was often followed into the bathroom by autograph seekers! I would hear them talking while I was in the stall. Things like: "Those are her shoes!"; "There she is!"; "Wait here, she'll be out in a minute"; "Oh my gosh, I'm peeing next to Miss America!"

The security detail that followed me made privacy all the more difficult to maintain, and I was amazed to learn how easily that security could be breached. One night, while on the road as Miss America, I woke to see a man—I think he was a member of the hotel staff—standing at the foot of my bed with a tray of drinks. I was sleepy, groggy, and stunned. I couldn't even move. I just sat up in bed and said, "What do you want?" The man couldn't speak English very well and stuttered that he was told to bring drinks to my room. I asked him to leave and told him that no one orders drinks at 1:30 A.M.!—certainly not for me. Thank God he turned and left when I told him to. I was scared to death. I never learned whether he was a poor waiter on an honest errand who had been sent to my room by some admirer, or who had been sent to my room by mistake, or was up to no good. But whatever he was doing, how in the world he had skirted security— especially given the extreme care the organization had taken to shelter and protect me—is really unbelievable. I've used the chain on my door ever since.

Another time a fire broke out in my hotel and I was stranded on the fire escape—with only my traveling companion Bonnie. No security in sight! Often, I had so much security that I had no privacy—and then, when something potentially dangerous really happened, I had none at all!

These experiences were some of the continual reminders that I just couldn't be a private person anymore, that people who met Miss America felt they had a right to participate in her life in a personal way. I guess that's part of the power of the crown. But I will say that even given all my Miss America dreams and all my experience in other pageants, I never fully understood just how the real experience would affect my private life.

In my case, I think the usual invasions of a Miss America's privacy became even greater because my battle with diabetes was so personal. There is such an emotional connection between diabetes and me, and between me as a spokeswoman for diabetes and others with the disease, as well as their friends and families. Because I was a prominent spokesperson about the disease, and because people felt they knew so much about me already, they also felt as though we were intimately associated. Because of this, I had unparalleled opportunities to be a role model, to encourage diabetes testing, and to raise money for research. But beyond a certain point, I needed a privacy barrier. I didn't want Nicole Johnson, as a person, to become a public commodity. But I was in the public eye so much—and still am, with a heavy schedule of public speaking—that I know that one (perhaps surprising) result of being Miss America is that I have become much more introverted. But it's been necessary in order to protect what little part of my life is still my own.

One way I coped with the lack of privacy was to retreat to the nearest restroom—when I wasn't followed. It was my hiding place. At functions I would excuse myself and then lock myself into a stall to read over my speech or jot down some thoughts for my talk. *Usually*, it was the only place that was quiet and where I was unlikely to be disturbed. Unless, of course, someone wanted an autograph. I suppose it would be sad, if it weren't so funny.

CHARITIES WITH CELEBRITIES

What kept me going when the inconveniences started to get to me was that I knew I was doing important work—work that I could not have done in any remotely comparable fashion had I not been Miss America. I thank God for the Miss America Organization and their trust in me to represent them. Whatever the frustrations, I was always grateful for this incredible opportunity.

I began my national speaking tour earlier in my reign than any other Miss America. My first stop was the Kmart Kids Race Against Drugs in Nashville, Tennessee. At the race, I found myself in a tractor racing against Kerry Strug, the Olympic gymnast. I guess tractor racing didn't require much athletic ability because I won the race!

After the race, it was time to be serious. I hit the road making speeches. I averaged two speeches a day and had no speechwriters. Typically my work days would consist of about six to seven hours of public appearances and meetings, plus at least an hour on the phone doing work with the Miss America office, and another hour or two on the computer writing speeches, responding to e-mail, or doing diabetes research. And that doesn't include travel—20,000 miles a month.

My first diabetes event was in Boston, Massachusetts, at an America's Walk for Diabetes with the American Diabetes Association. Executives from the ADA congratulated me on being *their* Miss America. I felt at home at this event. For the first time as Miss America I was doing the work that I believe God had been preparing me for all along. One of the most difficult things, I think, is trying to figure out God's plan or purpose for your life. Many people search their whole lives for it. Well, with God's grace, I had found my purpose—or at least an important part of it. In Psalm 32 it says: "I will instruct and teach you in the way you should go; I will counsel you and watch over you." I'd learned to listen for that quiet directing voice of conscience, and I'd learned to trust in God's plan.

Undeniably, the opportunity to see celebrities in the flesh at various charitable events was one of the most thrilling aspects of a thrilling year. My first star-studded event was the Carousel of Hope Ball in Los Angeles, an extravaganza held every two years to benefit diabetes research. To be honest, I was just as excited as anyone would be to meet celebrities at this event. Before the ball I decided to treat myself to a manicure and a pedicure, a luxury that I did not often enjoy. When they were finished, I had to make my way back to the hotel with wet fingers and toes. Fitted with only the best pedicurist's pink paper slippers, I sashayed across the street and into the beautiful Beverly Hills hotel. The hotel had actually rolled out a red carpet in preparation for the evening's event, and the press was already there. My curiosity got the best of me, and I had to see what else was being done to prepare for the event. So, I walked down the red carpet to the reception room in my jeans, T-shirt, and paper slippers. All the while, the press was congregating on both sides of the carpet—never knowing who I was! Such momentary anonymity was priceless—a fun victory over the people who kept me in a glass bowl.

The evening was phenomenal. I walked down the red carpet an hour later (this time dressed in a Rose Taft taupe lace gown) to meet a mass of photographers, flashing bulbs, and reporters screaming my name. Then it was off to the VIP reception room where all the stars were hanging out. I met them all: Kenny G, David Foster, Buzz Aldrin, President Ford, Betty Ford, Kate Jackson, Mary Hart, Mark Steines, Larry King, Roger Moore, Jackie Collins, Yasmine Bleeth, Richard Grieco, FloJo, Babyface, Quincy Jones, James Woods, Sly Stallone, Marlee Matlin, Celine Dion, Rod Stewart, Rachel Hunter, John Ratzenberger, Faith Ford, Jane Seymour, and more! I was so happy to be among them all in such a glamorous environment.

Dinner was next. I sat next to former president Gerald Ford. What do you talk to a president about? He was extraordinarily kind, gentle, and personable. On the other side of me were Angelica Houston and her husband. When I was called to the stage, Barbara Davis introduced me, and there I was in front of twelve hundred celebrities! I shared my story about what it's like to live life to the fullest with diabetes. The room was silent—for the first time all night! I couldn't believe that I was making an impact on this crowd. It was as though I commanded respect from them. Who would believe it?

I was on a roll. The very next night I attended the Make a Difference Day events taking place in Los Angeles. It was a lot of fun but far less glamorous than the ball I had attended the night before. Later, though, I went to a dinner party at the home of Hollywood heavyweights Barbara and Marvin Davis. What a house and what a guest list! The bathroom was as big as the living room in my old Virginia apartment, with a vanity along an entire wall. It had every type of expensive perfume you could imagine. At the dinner, each table had a gorgeous white chocolate horse centerpiece, and there was so much crystal and china for the place settings that it was easy to get lost among the cutlery. Everyone at the party was a

Hollywood power player of some kind—the people who *make* the stars. I was blown away at how many people came up to me complimenting me on my speech of the night before. One big-time producer even came up to me and said he would "be in touch." So movie people really did talk like that. (He never did get in touch.) Seated at my table were Danielle Steele, CoCo Chanel, and the Davises. I had Dom Perignon and caviar for the first time, but I didn't really care for either. Oh well, maybe I didn't fit in with the Hollywood crowd.

About one-third of the way through my term, I met President Carter and his wife, Rosalynn, at Super Bowl XXXIII in Miami. The former president was tremendously generous and gracious. They were both overwhelmingly kind. I cherish the photo that I have of the three of us. We spoke about their Habitat for Humanity project. Their example and willingness to give to others gave me extra motivation.

Unfortunately, before meeting President Carter, the Super Bowl events weren't that pleasant. My official NFL escort to one of the big Super Bowl bashes disappeared to hang out with his friends. I was left to wander around by myself with my traveling companion, which also left me without a dancing partner (Bonnie wasn't up for that duty, and I don't blame her). I guess even Miss America gets ditched every once in a while. Every American girl with boyfriend trouble should remember that—even Miss America gets the blues.

But that wasn't even the worst thing. During that Super Bowl weekend I was participating in a fashion show to benefit breast cancer when my shyness took over. All the other models were stars like Niki Taylor, Nancy O'Dell, Carmen Electra, Holly Robinson Peete, and Star Jones. I thought Nicole Johnson, Miss America, didn't quite fit in. After the show I met some of the sports stars who were also modeling at the event, including Sammy Sosa. As we were preparing to leave and go to yet another function, I was approached by one of Sammy's representatives. He said that Sammy wanted my telephone number and might like to see me again. Shocked, I told him that I didn't have a phone because I traveled too much. (I know. That was lame, but it's the only thing that came to mind.) The representative was persistent and pressed me for my hotel information. So that he would leave me alone, I politely told him that I would give him a business card (of course, my card didn't have any phone numbers on it, only a P.O. box). This so-called manager was so pushy that he even followed me into the women's dressing room as I went to retrieve a business card. I was amazed at this aggressive behavior. I know many women have experienced the feeling of not wanting to be asked out by somebody, but I thought this was just short of harassment. I did, however, get some huge bonus points with my brother for meeting Sammy Sosa.

A couple of days later, I spent one of my few attempted days off in San Antonio. After a morning-long conference call to the Miss America office about corporate sponsorships, I spent the afternoon browsing through a Mexican flea market. I bought a bracelet from a vendor who looked at me and said, "You look like one of those Miss America types, a model or star." I let him continue on and after a few moments of silence I asked, "Do you watch the pageant?" He looked at me apprehensively and said, "Well, I have seen it sometimes." Then he looked at me a little closer and said, "You've been in that, haven't you?"

"Uh-huh...I am her."

"Her who?"

"Miss America."

He gasped and then went around bragging to everyone that he had sold a bracelet to Miss America.

Soon after that I was on the *Donny and Marie Show* with John Ratzenberger (remember Cliff Clavin from *Cheers?*). It turns out his son has diabetes. Right before we went on the show he turned to me and, with tear-filled eyes, gave me a hug, telling me how much he appreciated my work and how much it meant to him to have someone like me as a role model for his son. That moment made my year. That's what it was all about. That's what motivates me to do what I'm doing. It wasn't the pursuit of the crown; it was using the crown to make a difference in people's lives.

I was sometimes able to use my newfound celebrity to make contact with people I would never have met otherwise. Shortly after I was first diagnosed, I bought a magazine about diabetes. Michelle McGann, the LPGA golf pro, was on the cover. One day while I was on the road as Miss America, Michelle called *me* to talk about my diabetes and about my using the pump. She explained that she had been diagnosed with diabetes many years before and that she used multiple daily injections of insulin to control the diabetes. She, like me, wanted better control and greater flexibility. She quizzed me about the pump, wanting to know how it *really* worked and what it was like living with the device. We talked for over an hour and really hit it off—there was an instant bonding between us. Shortly thereafter, she called me again, this time to tell me that she had decided to start using the pump! I was so excited that I was able to help her—it was as if I had a pump sister! We talked on and off for several months, and I would hear about her trying the pump on the golf course. We have remained friends for a few years now, and we try to see each other whenever we can. I was thrilled to be able to relate to someone who is high profile and dealing with the same issues I am. Her friendship is one of my treasures as Miss America—and as Nicole.

HITTING THE HEIGHTS

My activities as Miss America, albeit exhausting, were also exhilarating. Alex Noble once said, "Success is not a place at which one arrives but rather...the spirit with which one undertakes and continues the journey." I continued the journey throughout this great land. Being Miss America was definitely a phenomenal opportunity. It allowed me to pay off all of my college loans. It allowed me to speak on an issue that was and is terribly important to me. And it allowed me to see America—from New England to the Mississippi River to the Pacific Ocean.

In one of my most exciting adventures, a park ranger took me on a hike with his family to the top of Mount Rushmore. Ironically, a year later that park ranger's daughter was diagnosed with diabetes. You just never know.

There were other terribly emotional experiences. One came at a Navajo Indian Reservation in Tuba City, Arizona. It was heartbreaking to see such poor living conditions. We hear so much about the amount of government assistance Native Americans get, but from what I saw, the aid does not begin to meet the need. Everything was dirty and sandy. I stayed in the only hotel on the reservation. The hotel had a diner, and there was also a Taco Bell, a McDonald's, a Dairy Queen, and a liquor store. No wonder diabetes is rampant among the Native American population; their food options, at least where I visited, were so poor. I spoke at a high school to hundreds of children.

The children had been bused in from four states and several cities—just to hear about diabetes. My talk was well received, and, I believe, desperately needed. One of the great treasures I have is a photo of a girl who shared her ancient Navajo head-dress with me. We temporarily exchanged crowns that day.

Becoming Miss America changed my life forever. I hope I also changed the role of Miss America forever—from passive beauty queen to social activist. I was able to see beyond the glamour of winning the title and into the reality of what the title could accomplish. But I've always believed that "to whom much is given, much is required." I was given much, now I was destined to reach out. The crown was my passport to travel and touch others. The crown was my microphone. The crown was a representation of hope. And I did my best to spread that hope wherever I went. I still try to do so.

PART II: A PLAN FOR ACTION

"What do we live for if not to make life less difficult for each other?"
—GEORGE ELIOT

Chapter 9

QUEEN OF DIABETES

"Please God, no, not my brother!"

I was on the road as Miss America when I heard the news. I sat in the hotel room in Georgia, with tears streaming down my face. My brother had recently participated in a landmark research study, DPT-1, which was designed to detect the presence of Type I diabetes in at-risk individuals, specifically the siblings of young people with "juvenile" diabetes.

My brother, Scott, had tested positive; he, like me, had a genetic predisposition for diabetes. Never was I more concerned for anyone's health or future—not even my own. Soon, we found that Scott would need to undergo more tests. As it turns out, Scott never progressed to the "elite level," which would designate that he actually had the disease. I thank God for that—and for the medical knowledge that made these tests possible. It says in the book of Jeremiah: "But I will restore you to health and heal your wounds." I trust that God will allow my brother's hidden wound to heal.

I know some people are critical of medical trials. I even have a friend who doesn't want to have her children tested for fear of finding out that something *is* wrong or of becoming too neurotic a mother. She thinks that ignorance is bliss. Trust me, it isn't. Ignorance can mean ignoring the warning signs of diabetes and waiting until the condition turns deadly—as it almost did for me. Knowledge really is power—in this case, the power to save lives. And that's a commitment we should all make—especially when it comes to children.

WEARING THE CROWN . . . SHARING THE CROWN

Nothing was more important to me as Miss America than seeing the courage, and responding to the love, of children. One memory in particular is very special to me. While on the road one day between engagements, I received in the mail a crown made out of pink construction paper with the legend "QUEEN OF DIABETES" written across the bottom of it. It was from a little friend in New York State, a young boy named Brandon Witt who had himself been diagnosed with Type I diabetes. Despite my nonstop schedule of travel, speeches, lobbying, and appearances—which always left me with little time to "mind my manners"—I made sure to call him personally and thank him for that gift. This crown meant as much to me as my Miss America crown, because it represented the trust and faith of millions of children across the country.

Breaking with a tradition set by previous Miss Americas, I chose not to wear my crown to events or other appearances. I firmly believed that if the crown was on my head, then others couldn't touch it and feel its magic. By letting children see and handle the crown, I wished to instill in them the kind of healthy ambition necessary to see their dreams and aspirations realized. I wanted them to know that challenges in life—like diabetes—aren't roadblocks but stepping stones that empower us to rise to levels we couldn't achieve before. These challenges teach us perseverance, faith, trust, hope, respect for others, and empathy. By sharing my crown, I hoped to make it clear that they too could achieve whatever they set out to do.

Once, at an event during my year as Miss America, a little boy tried on the crown and looked in the mirror. I asked him what he wanted to be when he grew up, and he told me that he thought he wanted to be a movie producer but wasn't really sure. I told him to look in the mirror and say, "Yes, I can!" He repeated the words slowly and then went back to his family. About thirty minutes later, a man came up to me. He was sobbing. He was the boy's father, and he told me that for the first time his son told him that he felt he "could do something." It was so moving to see this child's self-esteem lifted and his father so encouraged, each transformed by the power of hope.

Other episodes soon gave me an even deeper appreciation of the responsibility that came with the title of Miss America. I remember vividly a talk I gave in Des Moines, Iowa, to the local Juvenile Diabetes Research Foundation chapter. As usual, there was a time set aside for questions and answers afterwards. In this case the children—all living with the challenge of diabetes—started to ask me question after question about my life with this disease. They seemed to want to know every detail about my personal struggle with "the monster": my highest blood sugar numbers; my lowest numbers; whether I had seizures like they sometimes did; whether I liked having diabetes. I realized that they desperately needed to identify their own pain and suffering, their own experience of isolation and loneliness with someone who seemed to be living a "normal" life, even a "glamorous" life. My ability to conquer my disease, at least to the extent that I could live my dream, gave them a reason for hope.

At that moment, I felt an awesome responsibility. One of the last questions asked by one of the children—a question I get from kids all over the country suffering from diabetes—was particularly poignant: "Miss America, will you find a cure for us?" Talk about awesome responsibility! But the truth is that this and similar questions always served to motivate me to do all I could during my time as Miss America (and since) to bring us closer to that goal. Seeing the trust and confidence that others placed in me helped me to recognize that I was not just fighting for myself, but for millions across the country for whom I was the most prominent spokesperson. I had to use my influence for those who had little influence themselves but were depending on me to be their voice. But I was inspired by *their* voices, *their* letters. Such as the letter I received from a beautiful young girl, who struggles, as I do, with Type I diabetes:

Dear Miss America,

Hello. My name is Marissa. I am eleven years old and I have diabetes, too. You are a very good example for young girls who have diabetes but are afraid that the disease will control their lives. Thank you for showing us that we can achieve any of our dreams, no matter who we are or what we have. I love to act and right now I am going to an acting camp. I also ride horses and really hope to compete in the Olympics someday. (And no one can stop me because of anything!) I play the cello, love art, and dance. I am really busy and my blood sugars are sometimes all over the place. I was diagnosed in September of 1997. My mom had

noticed the symptoms and took a urine sample to the pediatri-
cian. There was a lot of sugar in it and my mom picked me up
at school and I was at the hospital for about two days. I was really
nervous at first. I thought, "Oh no! I can't have any sugar any-
more!" But I discovered that that would not be the case at
all...I am in the fifth grade right now but school is going to end
in two days. I am off to middle school then! I am sad that I am
leaving my school because I really love it. I also love the nurse
there. She has been soooo wonderful since I got my diabetes. We
have become real buds. At first, I was the only one in the school
that had diabetes. But then my friend's little sister developed it
a few months ago. I have told her not to be scared and that it will
be OK. (She's only a first grader.) My mom also talked to her
mom. It feels nice knowing that you are helping someone out....
                                        Sincerely, Marissa

Marissa is vibrant, full of hopes and dreams, and is inspir-
ing other youngsters with the message that diabetes doesn't
have to slow you down. Marissa's mom is a hero, too. She had
her daughter tested. Thanks to that early diagnosis, Marissa
will continue to have a life full of activity, laughter, and
friends—and maybe even a trip to the Olympics someday.

TURNING PAIN INTO SOMETHING POSITIVE
"Mommy, why are you hurting me?" asks a little girl, looking
up at her mother with tears running down her face. It is the
same question every morning.

"I'm hurting you because I love you and because I want you
to grow up to be a strong, healthy, and active young woman,"
answers the mother with anguish in her heart as she gives her
precious child another insulin injection—an injection that is
keeping her two-year-old girl alive.

A seven-year-old boy, just diagnosed with diabetes, was at school playing on the playground when he realized none of the other children were playing with him. This went on for several days, until one day he mustered up enough courage in his little being to go over to the other kids and ask them, "Why won't you play with me?" The other children looked at him and said, "Our mommies and daddies say we can't play with you because we might catch diabetes."

These are but two of the thousands of real-life stories that cross my path every day. Letter after letter, story after story about how diabetes affects lives. Some are stories of hope, others of tragedy. I've had parents tell me they wake up three to four times a night to check their infant's blood sugar just to make sure their precious child will be alive in the morning. I never realized how many tears I would shed as Miss America—nor the level of passion that would well up in my heart and soul. There is nothing more precious than the innocence and the heart of a child. And when you see a disease like diabetes steal a child's innocence and break his heart, it is truly devastating. I've met many of the faces—children and parents—behind these stories, and they are the true motivation for my mission toward diabetes awareness—and one day a cure. I dream that my children will never know what the word diabetes means. And as the writer Sir James M. Barrie said, "Dreams do come true, if we only wish hard enough. You can have anything in life if you will sacrifice everything else for it."

BLOOM IN THE FACE OF ADVERSITY

Growing up is hard enough, but growing up with diabetes can be utterly demoralizing. The battle starts anew each morning. But aside from the strict daily regimen, the hardest part for some kids is trying to fit in when diabetes makes them feel as if they stand out. They don't want to admit that they are less perfect than or different from other kids. It is embarrassing having to leave early to go to the nurse or having to excuse yourself to go to the restroom.

One problem I've found, particularly with young people, is a resistance to wearing a medical ID for fear of being labeled. Many people see a medical ID, or an insulin pump for that matter, as a way for others to steal their identity or place them in a category. I say be proud of who and what you are. Why be ordinary?

But diabetes can carry with it a stigma to those who lack confidence or who have low self-esteem—and what kid hasn't felt a little uncertain or insecure at times? I share their frustration, because I share their disease. One mother told me that she can give her daughter all the financial help and love in the world, but I was able to give her child something more— hope. The little girl said, "Mommy, you don't understand, you don't live with this disease, but Nicole does." I am living proof that they don't have to be ashamed or feel alone—there are other people out there going through the same thing. Even for children, diabetes doesn't have to control their lives; they can control diabetes—and still be kids too.

I've been with many children and teens newly diagnosed with diabetes. And because I've been there, I know that a reassuring ear and a loving touch can break the ice, so I usually sit down and cry with them first, give them a hug, and tell them it's okay. Then I tell them that they can do anything they want to do. It doesn't matter that they have diabetes. It's just a roadblock—but they can go around it; they can find different paths. I talk about options they can choose in their medical management. Then I tell them what it's like for me, how I cope day in and day out. I tell them that they have to be strong—maybe it means making the tough choice not to eat the cupcakes at their friend's birthday party—but they can do it. They should never be ashamed of who they are, and they should never lose sight of their goals. They should make sure they are following their dreams, not someone else's, and then find the determination to make it happen.

Before the Miss America pageant, I learned an important philosophy, a philosophy that I have now adopted as one of my personal mottoes: *The flower that blooms in adversity is the most rare and most beautiful of all.* I took that to heart, and it became a kind of talisman throughout the competition.

When I finally made it to Miss Virginia, and later Miss America, I wanted everything about my performance to reflect the journey that had brought me there. It had been a tough road, but it was also filled with hope. While I sometimes wondered how I could overcome the obstacles I encountered, I never doubted that it was possible for me to succeed in life. I also knew that I had a message to share with the world. I felt discouraged and almost quit a few times, but I always knew in my heart that I could make it if I just tried a little harder. So I did, and I made it. And I tell children that they can, too. As the editor Michael Korda wrote, "To succeed, we must first believe that we can."

Some people like to be negative. They sometimes excuse it in the name of "realism." But diabetics—who have this one extra hurdle—can't afford to be negative or to listen to negative people. If you accept being told "no," if you give up, then you will never achieve anything. But if you refuse to give up, then it's impossible to fail. We need to remember the Biblical verse that says you have to run the race to completion, but God will help you, He will be by your side, and will be your lamp post and the wings affixed to your shoes.

CROWNING THE REAL HEROES

The year I gave up my title, less than twenty-four hours before I would crown the next Miss America, I rode on the Miss America float for the legendary Atlantic City boardwalk parade. I was so gratified to see crowds of people holding up signs that read: "Thank you Miss America 1999 from the sixteen million other Americans with diabetes"; "Thanks for helping us get pumps!"; "We're Pumpers like you"; and "Thank you Miss America!" I saw people waving black boxes in the air—at first I couldn't make out what they were. Then it hit me: they were insulin pumps, and these people were thanking me for making them aware of this liberating invention for those who suffer from diabetes. As I stood there on the float in my jeweled gown, tears ran down my cheeks as the realization dawned that all the travel, all the stress, all the speechifying had been worth it. There were kids on the parade route with signs that read: "Nicole, We're pumped up too!" and "Miss America, I'm just like you" with photos of needles and pumps.

That was gratifying—and so was becoming an honorary Pump Girl! "The Pump Girls" are a group of four southern California teenagers who met at a camp and began singing together. The head of the Pediatric Adolescent Diabetes Research and Education Foundation was so impressed by "The Pump Girls" that she introduced them to a music producer who gave them a recording deal. Since then, they've been touring the country, giving hope to other kids. These girls are proof: you can have diabetes and still have an impact on society—you can even become a pop sensation!

That's really the whole point—making diabetes an issue that is popularly understood. That's my goal, and to that end I've not only given speeches and granted interviews, I've autographed everything from car tires to glucose monitors and insulin pumps. Once, as part of a diabetes fundraiser, I even consented to be auctioned—the prize was lunch with me the next day! I stood in the middle of the ballroom floor as people were bidding on me. The auctioneer called out, "Going once...going twice...sold for $2,000!" The winners were a dear family with two young teenage boys—both had diabetes. I went over to say hello and was greeted by the mother who said, "You were worth a lot more!"

As part of the prize package, we were to ride in a limousine to a fancy restaurant. The boys told me that they really didn't want to go to the fancy restaurant—they wanted to go through the drive-through at McDonald's. So away we went to McDonald's in our limo. The only problem was that we didn't fit through the drive-through, so we went inside, ordered, and took our takeout to the car. Then the boys wanted me to go to their basketball game—so we did! What a treat—I had never done anything like that before. We arrived at the school and both boys proudly escorted me into the gym. I played basketball with them and the team during warm-ups—in a suit and heels! The team was really impressed when Miss America made a basket. I decided not to press my luck, and quit while I was ahead. The families in the gym were so excited and delighted that I would come to their game, but I don't think they knew how much they brightened *my* life that day.

I often think of these fun-loving boys, "The Pump Girls," and the sign-waving friends along the parade route. I remember every hospital I've visited, every hand I've held, every person's story I've heard. They have all taught me irreplaceable lessons—not only about overcoming adversity, but about giving and what giving can do. And also about the definition that Ernest Hemingway gave to courage: grace under pressure.

I remember one young girl, in particular, who demonstrated that grace. I was speaking at a health fair in Birmingham, Alabama. It was a hot, steamy day, and I was perspiring just sitting at a table signing autographs (there are some days that are just too hot even for us southern girls!). There were a number of people lined up in front of my table, including one teenage girl who was waiting patiently for an autograph. I looked up and couldn't help but notice she was very white and was starting to sway. I glanced at her after signing another autograph and saw her suddenly collapse. Several of us rushed over to help her. It was a good thing that she was wearing a medic ID that said she was a diabetic because we immediately knew what was wrong—she was paralyzed with a low blood glucose level. Several people ran off to get her some lemonade.

I knew exactly what she was feeling, since I'd had this happen to me. I sat on the floor with her for a few minutes to make sure that she felt comfortable and wasn't embarrassed. It is hard at any age to have this happen to you, but the teen years are such a delicate time. We talked about funny experiences with lows until she relaxed enough to get her blood glucose back to normal. But she handled herself so well, with a natural poise that I could only envy. She smiled as I helped her up and thanked me with a hug. I was glad to be there for her—and I was glad to witness her grace under pressure.

RULES TO LIVE BY

On many of the stops I made as Miss America, I talked about my rules for living:

Wake up, show up, and pay attention. Make sure you get up and get going *every day.* Don't give in to self-pity or self-doubt. As H. Jackson Brown Jr. said: "Opportunity dances with those who are already on the dance floor."

Love something, particularly yourself. Accept yourself. Believe in your heart that you're not a damaged individual.

Never give up. Refuse to give up and you cannot fail.

Once, I talked about my rules at a children's hospital in Phoenix. On a return visit to Phoenix, almost a year later, a few of those same kids came to visit *me.* This time they brought their doctors who told me what a difference my previous visit had made in the care of those youngsters. Experiences like that really put life in perspective. I was humbled—and happy to have helped. To be honest, I was stunned that I had made such an impact on their lives.

Part of my message, for all people, but especially children and their parents, is one of education, but the other is one of hope. Education, discipline, and determination can help parents and children overcome the difficulties of diabetes.

Another anecdote illustrates the importance of education and awareness. In the spring of 1999, I was interviewed by an Indianapolis TV station. During that interview I described the signs and symptoms of diabetes. A young mom was watching the program and realized that her toddler was experiencing those very signs. She took her little girl to the hospital where she was diagnosed with diabetes. Recently I had the privilege of meeting that mother and her beautiful, rambunctious little girl (now happily controlling her diabetes) who is not more than four years old. Her family e-mailed me after our meeting:

> *Lori and I would like to thank you for spending time with Lindsay. You are a great role model for her. We've wanted you to know how your diabetes education has affected our lives and mostly Lindsay's. Seeing you on television two years ago gave Lori and I the first clues to her diagnosis. That is something that we will never forget. We thank you. Lindsay thanks you. Continue to fight the good fight. If you need a quick boost in energy, you can stop by Indianapolis and spend some time with Lindsay again. When we got home tonight Lindsay said, "My heart is full of joy" and "I miss Nicole." She also wanted to know if you could come to her house to play. We will email again later, after Lindsay gets her very own Mini-Med!*
>
> *God Bless, Bob, Lori, and Lindsay*

More recently they wrote me to tell me she was participating in a research trial and had started using the insulin pump:

> *Hello! Just a note to let you know that Lindsay received her "real" pump yesterday. We are all very excited. She is doing great and adjusting very well. She wore a dummy pump for about one month and would remind us if we wouldn't put it on her. She is very excited that her pump is blue just like yours. Thank you for spending time with her and for being such a wonderful role model for everyone with diabetes. She will be in the pump study for one year from yesterday, then she will be able to have her very own pump. We are so thankful for how well she has adapted and know that part of that is because you were so kind to show her yours.*

GETTING INVOLVED

I met an especially brave family one snowy day in Iowa at a Juvenile Diabetes Research Foundation walkathon. (The walkathon is the third largest fundraiser for JDRF in the nation.) This family really hit home with me because they had participated in the same DPT-1 trial that had diagnosed my brother Scott as having a genetic predisposition to diabetes. DPT-1 involves patients with Type I diabetes and their first-degree relatives; a small percentage of this group is at an increased risk of developing diabetes because of a genetic predisposition. Since early detection and prevention are so important, this trial represents all that is best in the treatment of my disease.

In this family, the eldest two children have diabetes, and the youngest tested positive for the antibody. The family was devastated. But after that initial shock, the mom went on to dedicate her life to fighting the disease and working for her children and their future. She was the organizer of the walk and also was the local JDRF representative. She turned the pain of this disease into a positive force in the fight against diabetes.

As I continued to meet thousands of children with diabetes in my travels, it occurred to me that I needed to leave them with something more personal than the standard autographed picture of Miss America—something they could carry with them in their heart. I devised a secret handshake only for kids with diabetes called the "pinky promise" which I did with each of the children. Locking pinkies, I asked them to promise that they would always take care of their diabetes; that they would always let others help them with their diabetes; and that they would never give up on themselves or their medical condition. Each pledge was followed by a solemn "I promise" from both of us. It was a way of making them realize that they are special—and that diabetes doesn't have to defeat dreams.

While at that walkathon kickoff event in Iowa, a little girl pulled my pant leg saying, "Miss America? Miss America?"

She asked me if I had seizures like she did and asked if my lows hurt. "Miss America, how can I make them not hurt?" she asked.

The only way I can think to make it not hurt is for more of us to care for our children with testing, education, and love. My experiences have brought home to me the absolute importance of caring support from family and friends. That support is as vital to any diabetic as insulin or oxygen.

Once in Denver at an event for the Barbara Davis Center for Diabetes and the Children's Diabetes Foundation, several mothers of children with diabetes approached me with questions about marriage. What was the probability of their child finding a lifelong mate who was sensitive, compassionate, and understanding enough to cope with the situation of a spouse with diabetes? Was it unrealistic even to hope for someone to commit to a relationship with a diabetic? Usually in the "question and answer" period that follows most of my speaking engagements, I feel pretty confident, self-possessed, and prepared to answer any questions, if only because of all the practice I've had. But this time I was completely at a loss; I really had no idea how to answer. In my own case, I always believed that God would just send me the right man at the right time, but this hardly seemed like an adequate answer to the very realistic concerns expressed by these mothers. I told them that I realized how important these questions were and related the story of how one former boyfriend's mother had been particularly insensitive in her comments, cautioning him against me when she became aware that I had diabetes. But other than commiserating, I didn't really have an answer for them.

In the time since, I've given those comments a lot of consideration. I began to wonder: Would I really find the right man? Was it really possible that some generous soul could commit to a lifetime with me—as well as my diabetes, which is a part of who I am? For whoever it is, it will be a step into the unknown and a real risk. I worry sometimes about various issues related to marriage: that I will be a burden to my future husband; about children and the pain I would feel if my child were diagnosed with this condition. There's no way to predict the future. I do rest assured that when I get married, my husband will care more about my diabetes than any other part of my life—as if my diabetes were also his condition. He will want me to be with him, and healthy, for many, many years to come, and he will understand that in order to achieve that goal we must fight diabetes together. I guess that's what's meant by "for better or worse." The important thing—for anyone who takes marriage seriously—is to find someone who really means those words.

Diabetes is not a one-person disease. The person living with it has the ultimate power, but that person also needs support and love—and action—from everyone. This is a disease we can change. The statistics are reversible if we continue to be vocal advocates and educators. We can give children with diabetes hope for a brighter tomorrow. Apathy does not produce results—planning, persistence, and a positive attitude do!

And if you are a young person with diabetes, don't let diabetes stop you. Don't let diabetes hold you back. I encourage you to bloom in the face of your adversity. You can accomplish any goal and be anything you want to be. The control rests in your hands. When you gain control of your life (blood sugars included), you not only make a difference in your own well-being, but you enable yourself to make a difference in the life of someone else. Other people who are struggling will be motivated and inspired by your success and will have something to strive for. When they know that there is no limit to what they can do by seeing what you have done, you have given them the greatest gift of all. I know that diabetes can be difficult to adjust to—because I had to adjust to it, too, and it wasn't easy. But if we all keep striving forward (and keep testing our blood sugars), one day we'll beat this—together.

Chapter 10

THE POLITICS OF DIABETES

"What's your favorite color?"

It was at the press conference immediately after I won the title. I was prepared to start my tenure as Miss America by talking about my plans to use my crown—and the celebrity that goes with it—to serve society by promoting diabetes awareness. Instead, a reporter covering the press conference felt compelled to ask a question that was better suited for the dating game. It seemed designed to play to the caricature of the air-headed beauty queen with nothing intelligent to say.

I was appalled. As someone with a master's degree in journalism who has always taken her intellectual development seriously, I was also personally insulted. With my reporting experience, I knew that this reporter had not taken his assignment seriously. He was attempting to make a mockery of the whole thing: of all that I had been fighting to achieve, of all the adversity I had overcome.

I paused for a minute to gain my composure, then looked the journalist squarely in the eye and said, "If you all don't have anything important to ask me, let me tell you what I'm going to do with my term and my year as Miss America." I then talked about my plan to raise diabetes awareness. I still remember the applause that swept across the room after I was finished.

It was an important moment, perhaps the defining moment of my tenure as Miss America. I had taken a hostile, sarcastic question and turned it into an opportunity to talk about something positive. A very wise man once said, "Don't waste your energy and your time—which belong to God—throwing stones at the dogs that bark at you on the way. Ignore them." I've taken that advice to heart.

One of my primary goals as Miss America was to campaign for greater investment in diabetes research and prevention. While money is certainly not the only measure of success, I think it says a lot that during the time I held the title, more money was raised for diabetes research than had—or has—been raised for the cause of any other Miss America.

As Miss America, I realized that I had to use the "bully pulpit" of my position to get my message out through the mass media—which is the only place that most people get their information. In the last analysis, that means knowing how to work the media and keep them focused on the message that you want to talk about instead of what they would like you to talk about. In public relations, that's called "staying on message," and it's all important for anyone in the position of a spokesperson.

How many times have we heard phrases like, "If you eat too much candy, you'll wind up with diabetes." Or, "He's got everything under control; he may not exercise much, but he always takes his insulin on schedule." Or, "Diabetes might be important but it's not a looming health crisis like AIDS." These were the myths I wanted to bust.

Unfortunately, as we all know, the press is usually more interested in controversy and sensationalism than in accurately relating the content of what someone in the spotlight says. I came to understand this very quickly as Miss America.

CREATING CONTROVERSY

Occasionally, when someone brings up an issue that's either embarrassing or irrelevant to what you'd like to say, it's best just to ignore the question. Once backstage before a television appearance, the Reverend Jesse Jackson made a derogatory comment to me about being "the one who won the bathing suit competition." I was horrified that such a prominent public figure would make such a shallow remark. But instead of getting angry, I figured I would fill in the blanks. I started talking about my message, "I am on a national speaking tour promoting the important issue of..."

But sometimes it is impossible to "stay on message" if your questioner is determined to talk about irrelevancies. I had to cut short a radio appearance in mid-interview when it became apparent that the interviewer was only interested in being crude and talking about sexuality, which I consider to be a private matter inappropriate for public discussion. At times like this, standing up for your beliefs—even if it's difficult at the moment—wins you a great deal more than it costs.

Even after I gave up the title in September 1999, the media's appetite for controversy did not die down. During the Republican Party convention that nominated George W. Bush in August of 2000, I accepted a request for an interview from C-SPAN, the cable television channel that provides twenty-four-hour coverage of political events. I thought it might provide an opportunity to talk about my work with diabetes and even perhaps why I supported the Republican candidate for president.

Several months previous to this, George W. Bush had accepted an invitation to speak at Bob Jones University in Greenville, South Carolina. Former presidents, including Ronald Reagan and George W.'s father, as well as countless other politicians, had spoken at the conservative Christian school. I knew George W. Bush regarded his appearance there as unremarkable. It was another chance to speak to the conservative Christians who constitute an important part of his constituency. The media—and rival candidates—soon turned his appearance into an endorsement of the school's policies, which had included banning interracial dating among students.

When I appeared on C-SPAN, the controversy—which had occurred some months before—had ceased to be news. But the interviewer—perhaps making a link between Bob Jones and my alma mater, Regent, which has a reputation as a conservative Christian university—brought up the subject anyway, asking for my views on interracial dating.

I said that everyone should be free to date whomever they like, and I would never sit in judgment on anyone's decision.

He asked me directly if I would date a person of another race. I told him that was not my preference. I gave my personal opinion based on a personal decision; my stated preference had nothing to do with any general belief on the subject. Some men would not find me at all attractive because I don't have blonde hair. I don't think that makes them bigots. I strongly support inclusion—as I made clear on the same program—and equal rights for all. I am strongly against racism or racial profiling. I also have a policy never to lie or falsify answers when asked directly.

I probably should have known better. Personal honesty and sincerity have never been virtues that are always valued very highly by the media. A few days later, a news website tried to create a controversy out of my remarks. Under a banner that blared "Former Miss America Gets Ugly," it summarized my comments as follows: "Basically she is saying that everyone can do what they wish, but for her, she judges people by the color of their skin." Another lesson in how you can't let yourself get diverted from your message.

KNOWLEDGE IS POWER

Staying on message is important—because the message is the issue.

It took so long for me to get diagnosed because none of us, not me, not my parents, not my friends, not even some of the doctors I had seen, were looking for it. How could everyone miss it? Well, one reason is that none of us knew what to look for—or even that we should be looking for anything. We were completely in the dark, which is why diabetes is so often called the hidden or silent killer. I want to make sure that it's not hidden any longer. I want people to know just how prevalent diabetes is—and how important it is to catch it in the early stages.

One small step in the direction of a greater awareness of the costs that diabetes inflicts on our society is the Diabetes Awareness Stamp, issued by the United States Post Office on March 16, 2001. Only the third medical-related stamp issued by the government, the stamp bears the legend "Know More

About Diabetes." It was gratifying to see something I had been working for since my time as Miss America finally come to fruition. If it inspires just one person to educate himself about diabetes—a decision that could literally save that person's life—it was worth it.

Each year Americans spend more than a hundred *billion* dollars to treat diabetes and its complications. Every forty seconds someone is diagnosed with the disease. Someone dies from it every three minutes. It strikes regardless of age, race, or sex.

THE SEARCH FOR THE MISSING MILLIONS

In fact, millions of Americans today are walking around totally ignorant that they have diabetes. While over eleven million have been diagnosed with the disease, at least six million Americans are living at risk every day because their diabetes is undiagnosed.

In 1999, during my year as Miss America, my Search for the Missing Millions Campaign sponsored by Eli Lilly found 640 people with undiagnosed diabetes. That number might seem small, but that was from a screening of just ten thousand people. In other words, 6 percent of the people we tested had undiagnosed diabetes. These people had no idea that they were seriously ill.

On one occasion after a speech, a woman came to me with tears running down her face. She told me that her mother had had diabetes but that due to her shame and embarrassment about her condition, she had told no one about it—until it was too late. Even her family did not suspect how ill she really was. This poor woman died needlessly because she was afraid to reveal a medical condition that she bore little—or no—responsibility for acquiring. It struck her—as it struck me—like a mugger in the night.

In the absence of diagnosis and proper treatment, a hidden diabetic is in danger of blindness, kidney failure, amputation, and even death. A person with diabetes may appear healthy and well, but that person is two to four times more likely than a healthy person to suffer a heart attack or stroke. This year alone, hundreds of thousands of people in this country will die of diabetes-related causes, and too often these deaths could have been prevented with proper treatment. The search for these "missing millions" is on—and we have no time to lose.

THE DIABETES EPIDEMIC

Scientific research continues to play a major role in finding treatments for diabetes and will someday find a cure. But much more has to be done—and quickly. Diabetes is striking our country in epidemic proportions. Recent studies have reported a dramatic increase in Type II diabetes among children and teenagers, which is highly unusual. Young people, age thirty and under, are most often diagnosed with Type I diabetes—the type that afflicts only 5 to 10 percent of all those with the disease. The far more common form, Type II diabetes, usually attacks adults in their late forties and older.

While we don't know for sure why Type II diabetes is skyrocketing in epidemic numbers, it seems to be connected to a sedentary lifestyle and eating high calorie foods. In plain English, people are getting fatter. In fact, obesity is now thought to trigger between 50 and 75 percent of the new cases of Type II diabetes in this country. And as the spread of Type II in young people has shown, children with unhealthy lifestyles—children who eat fatty foods and watch TV and play computer games instead of playing outside—are also at serious risk.

From my experience, I know that all it takes is a single touch to want to get involved to reverse these numbers. Hold the hand of a child stricken with diabetes and you'll know why I'm committed to doing everything I can to help find a cure.

I am not, obviously, a research scientist, a medical doctor, or a trained nurse. But what I do with my own gifts enhances theirs. During World War II, Winston Churchill coined the phrase, "Give us the tools, and we will finish the job." Well, as Miss Virginia and Miss America I knew I could help deliver the tools to the scientists, doctors, and nurses. I could raise awareness about this deadly disease; I could be the ambassador for the over sixteen million Americans—diagnosed and undiagnosed—who have it. I could help raise money for the research, clinics, and care that can defeat diabetes.

Some who taught me by example just what kind of impact a title winner can have in this respect is Michelle Kang, Miss Virginia from 1996, who has become one of my best friends. Michelle's platform issue was the prevention of child abuse. She inspired the way I approach my work with diabetes; the way she was so passionate in her advocacy of her issue encouraged me to show the same kind of heart in the way I talked about diabetes. There was also Heather Whitestone, Miss America 1995, who didn't let her hearing loss get in the way of her goals. She showed me that no circumstance dictates a person's ability to succeed. I'm certain that passion is one of the keys to my success as an advocate for my own issue.

GETTING INVOLVED

Diabetes is a political issue because so much funding for medical research comes from the government. I know a lot of Americans are afraid of politics or dislike it. They see the word *politics* and they run. But you shouldn't. I've seen what the political process can do. It can change lives—for the better. And if we're not involved in politics, others—who don't have the right priorities—will have a monopoly on political power and influence.

This is definitely the case with medical research funding. For example, between 1980 and 1996—when the death rate from diabetes increased by 30 percent—National Institutes of Health spending on diabetes research *dropped* by 30 percent, relative to their total budget. While the situation has improved in subsequent years, funding for diabetes research still doesn't come close to reflecting the enormous social costs of diabetes compared to other diseases.

While I would never want to pit one disease against another in a battle over limited research dollars, it only makes sense to ask whether our money is being spent wisely, on the things that constitute the greatest threats to public health. The diabetes epidemic, especially Type II, is increasing at an alarming rate. Since 1990, all categories of diabetes have increased by 41 percent. They have increased 70 percent among thirty- to thirty-nine-year-olds. Diabetes afflicts more Americans, kills more Americans, and costs America more money than AIDS and breast cancer combined. But for every dollar the government spends trying to cure diabetes, it spends seven dollars trying to cure AIDS and breast cancer.

The fact is that politics, lobbying, and public awareness are necessary to get the appropriate funding to fight any disease. Funding for diabetes research has always lagged behind funding for more trendy diseases because of a lack of public awareness. The lobbies for increased spending on AIDS and breast cancer research are disciplined special interest groups.

Ironically, diabetes doesn't have the same political clout precisely because it doesn't have a politicized "interest group."

I realized that my first priority as a volunteer lobbyist and fundraiser was to act as the "public face" of diabetes, using my talents as a communicator to help both the public and their representatives in Congress recognize the human suffering—and lost human potential—behind the statistics. I also had to point out what often speaks loudest to politicians—the financial cost. Diabetes is a significant cause of both heart disease and stroke (the first and third leading causes of death in the United States), which together cost our nation about $218 billion a year. It's the leading cause of kidney disease, which costs an additional $40 billion each year. That's all in addition to the over $100 billion that diabetes alone costs our society in treatment, disability, and mortality.

The conclusion is inescapable: money invested in diabetes research, prevention, and education *now* will result in enormous savings—both in terms of medical costs and human lives—in the future. Politicians also need to understand that the prospects for rapid and exciting research advances to fight diabetes are incredibly promising. But politicians tend to think in terms of short-term outlays rather than long-term savings. As former House Speaker Newt Gingrich stated on *Good Morning America* in 1994:

> [W]e don't today pay for training you, as a diabetic, how to take care of yourself. We will pay to put you in the hospital [and to] amputate your leg when you fail to take care of yourself. But literally, the government bias today is to not pay for the preventive and educational experience that will lower your costs.

Unfortunately, that situation still persists. We would go a long way towards eliminating the $45 billion a year the federal government spends on diabetes treatment and care if more were invested in research and prevention. And it's not just a matter of educating politicians. Despite the fact that treating diabetes is so expensive, insurance companies and health management organizations have been slow to cover preventive care and as a result are costing themselves a bundle in expenses for diabetes related illnesses.

Another big obstacle is that politicians favor across-the-board spending increases that seem fair but that in reality fail to respond to new developments in research or diagnosis. The number of people with diabetes is exploding faster than any other major disease, yet you wouldn't know that from the funding diabetes receives. In 1999 alone, diabetes in the United States rose by about 6 percent in what the government itself calls an "unfolding epidemic." When you have an epidemic on your hands, politics as usual won't work.

GETTING THE JOB DONE

It was a special moment for me in January 1999 when, as Miss America, I saw legislation enacted in Richmond, Virginia, that I'd been helping to push for three years. We achieved significantly broader insurance coverage for state employees with diabetes, covering supplies (such as syringes, test strips, and monitors) as well as self-management education—the first step toward coverage for all citizens. Moments before the final vote at the state house, I was granted the privilege of addressing the legislators. It was my great honor to be only the third guest of the Virginia Senate—after Al Gore and Margaret Thatcher—to be allowed to speak from the Senate floor.

There I was, in the building designed by Thomas Jefferson, which has housed Virginia lawmakers for two centuries; which had seen Robert E. Lee vested with the command of all Virginia forces in the War Between the States; which had seen the election of the first black governor in the South. Now I had my own opportunity to express my thanks to the lawmakers who were in the process of writing a new page of Virginia history.

The only political experience that surpassed that thrill was when I officially launched my Miss America platform on the steps of the United States Capitol in October 1998. It was the earliest and most successful launch in the history of the Miss America Organization to date. In addition to my speech, the event included remarks from Speaker Newt Gingrich and Senator John Warner, among many other luminaries. More than two hundred legislators had signed on to support my initiative.

It was probably the greatest honor and greatest moment of my life. When I finished speaking, even cynical members of the press had tears in their eyes, as did many of the politicians, some of whom had a personal connection to the disease. Before the press conference, I had the opportunity to meet with Speaker Gingrich in his office. Speaker Gingrich picked up the phone and called his mother-in-law, a woman who inspired him to speak out on behalf of diabetes because of her personal battle with the disease. His gesture taught me a lot about the personal factors that contribute to the advocacy of a cause.

Along with all the seriousness of politics and lobbying, there is also a fair share of humor. In March of 1999, I was back on Capitol Hill for the American Diabetes Association's annual Rally for a Cure. To my surprise, it was held in the midst of a massive snowstorm. Having grown up in Florida and Virginia Beach, this was the last thing I expected in the spring, and I showed up in open-toed black heels. Big mistake. When it was over, my feet were half frozen. With the camera crew from ABC's *20/20* in tow (they were there to cover the event), I went inside the Capitol Building ladies room to use the hand dryer to thaw out my feet. A "behind the scenes" look at Miss America that most people probably never expected to see—feet propped up on the Capitol's bathroom wall under a hand dryer—and might never want to see again. Chalk it up to the perils of public life.

Actually, the fact that all these thousands of people, some from great distances, were attending a rally in the middle of a snowstorm in mid-March made the event all the more meaningful. Ultimately, the best thing about the rally was that it encouraged people to talk to their legislators about diabetes. It was because of the rally that I was able to meet with Speaker Hastert and the House Appropriations Committee. Call it fate, or perhaps just a fluke, but the committee was actually meeting in the Speaker's office when I visited, and it invited me in to say "hello." Needless to say, I took the opportunity to "work the room," as Hastert mentioned admiringly when I left. It was a fruitful meeting, but I have to say it was a blow no longer having a high-profile, personal advocate like former Speaker Gingrich, who was so passionate about the issue.

WALKING THE HALLS OF POWER

Lobbying can be both frightening and exhilarating—but in either case, you can make a big impact in the way a congressman or senator thinks about an issue. It is all a little overwhelming at first, especially because you feel as if your voice is just one among millions of people who want to be heard. After a while, though, you begin to realize that members of

Congress don't hear from their constituents as much as you might think. Sometimes, just a handful of citizens can make a tremendous difference in the way a member looks at, feels about, or votes on a particular issue. A state senator in Virginia once told me that it only takes five phone calls or letters to catch her attention, because she and her colleagues consider that type of response on a single issue to be a groundswell. Senator Susan Collins from Maine became involved with this issue of diabetes as a result of a single visit by a constituent and her family who came to talk with her about their problems with diabetes and access to proper care. Collins decided to do some research, and today she is one of the most vocal advocates of diabetes awareness and research, as well as cochair of the Senate Diabetes Caucus.

So, your influence as a voter, constituent, or lobbyist is much more significant than it might appear at first glance. You don't need to be a noted authority on an issue to call, write, or visit a legislator. The key is to be professional, know your subject, be able to talk about it anecdotally, get to know the key staffers on a personal level, and follow through on your promises. Here are some other tips:

BE ON TIME. You can never overestimate the importance of punctuality. When you are late for an appointment, it is not only an indication that you are disorganized and scatter-brained, it also sends the message that you don't regard the person you're meeting with very highly. It is an inconvenience for others and, on top of that, it is downright rude. On the other hand, if you are always prompt—or even a bit ahead of time—it sends the message that you are in control and have everything together, and that you respect the time commitment of the person you're meeting with.

HAVE A PLAN. It's usually best not to improvise your way through a presentation or even an informal meeting. You should have an agenda of what you would like to talk about, particular points you would like to get across, even anecdotes you would like to use. This doesn't mean you'll be reading from note cards the whole time (one note card with a *few* notes might help), but it does mean having a handle on how you want to communicate your issue, rather than relying on pure inspiration.

DO YOUR HOMEWORK. It may seem like an obvious point, but it's really important to know what you're talking about. Unless people see that you have a thorough knowledge of your subject matter, your appeals will be dismissed. You have to make a good case and have strong answers for tough questions. If people sense that you're winging it, or that your knowledge of a problem is superficial, it doesn't bode well for your proposed solution.

KEEP IT SHORT AND SIMPLE. People are busy. Just because a person consents to meet with you doesn't mean you should feel free to waste his or her time by being long-winded. It's important to keep things concise and to the point; going on diatribes or trying to show your encyclopedic knowledge of a subject is counterproductive, and usually impossible to follow. On the other hand, if you make a few, well-chosen points, and reiterate them in a memorable way, they are likely to stick in the minds of your listeners.

PAY ATTENTION TO CURRENT ISSUES BEFORE CONGRESS. If you come across as only being interested in advancing your own agenda, you may not get very far. It helps a lot to show a genuine interest in how your issue fits into the big picture of congressional politics. Know what the key issues are for your congressman and what motivates his political philosophy. Doing this research is important in knowing how best to communicate your case.

PREPARE A STATEMENT PAPER TO LEAVE FOR THE MEMBER AND THE STAFF. Since most professionals talk to many people every day, it's a good idea to leave behind some documentation of the meeting that will serve as a reminder and reference about your issue. Leave a short, pithy summary of your agenda.

BE POLITE. Manners matter. You can know your issue thoroughly but lose your case through lack of social graces. It's not that difficult: smile, be gracious, avoid being defensive or obnoxious, and don't lose your cool. Attractive "packaging" goes a long way toward winning people over to your point of view.

WRITE A "THANK YOU" NOTE. An important part of manners is displaying your gratitude. It's amazing how many people don't bother to do this. That extra little detail of following up your meeting with a personal note of thanks means a lot—not least because it doesn't happen every day. And it should be a personal note, not a form letter that shows about as much consideration as the Internal Revenue Service. People will be impressed that you took the time to show your thanks, and that will influence how they view both you and your agenda.

GETTING RESULTS

These guidelines worked for me. In 1999 and 2000, I was able to help boost funding for the National Institutes of Health, help pass diabetes-related legislation in close to half a dozen states, and work with state legislatures to improve insurance coverage for millions of people with diabetes.

Mind you, I didn't score a brilliant success every time. One of my worst experiences was a meeting with Dr. Harold Varmus, then director of the National Institutes of Health. I had been warned beforehand that Dr. Varmus was quite intimidating. But it was worse than I feared. First, he refused to meet with anyone but me, even though we had suggested that the meeting include representatives of the American Diabetes Association. Then, he proceeded to tell me that although my work with diabetes was wonderful, I would not see any of my funding goals realized because there were more pressing issues affecting a greater number of people. He talked about not pigeonholing National Institutes of Health funding. His whole tone was patronizing; it felt more like a lecture than a meeting. I got the impression that he didn't want "amateurs" dictating National Institutes of Health funding. That was for him to decide. If you lobby for an issue, you'll find plenty of "turf warriors" like Dr. Varmus.

Still, while a great deal was accomplished in terms of *public* funding for diabetes research and education during my time as Miss America, the private sector has vital initiatives of its own. One example is the "Search for the Missing Millions" campaign sponsored by Eli Lilly and Company. More than six million Americans are living at risk every day because their diabetes is undiagnosed. Millions of them have blood sugar levels that are out of control—symptoms that are seriously damaging their health and are potentially fatal. The "Search" uses diabetes screening to find these missing millions. Another example is Lilly's current diabetes awareness program called "Peaks and Valleys." This initiative educates patients, medical professionals, and health care providers about hyperglycemia, hypoglycemia, and postprandial (after meal) glucose levels—the "peaks and valleys" of life with diabetes.

Other private sector companies sponsoring diabetes related programs include Minimed, Roche, and Bristol Myers Squibb. In fact, there was more corporate sponsorship of the Miss America program and my platform during my year than ever before. Over the last three years, I've helped generate more than $14 million in contributions from private sources for diabetes research—a fact I'm extremely proud of, because that means we're $14 million closer to a cure.

Getting involved is easy, but I'll confess staying involved takes effort. It takes commitment. But it's worth it when you think of how many people you can help—and how many lives can be saved.

LEADING BY EXAMPLE

I try to teach by personal example. All the eloquence in the world can't match the power of practicing what you preach, of taking responsibility for your life and taking hold of your own destiny. During my year as Miss America, I developed a close friendship with a wonderful woman at the Juvenile Diabetes Research Foundation named Jane Adams. In her early thirties, she became one of my role models. She and I talk often about our shared condition and try to challenge and motivate each other to excellence.

Through the example of my newfound freedom in monitoring and dosing with the insulin pump, she decided to start the pump herself. Not only was I able to instill in her the self-confidence she needed to overcome her fears and dependence, but I helped inspire her to make a decision that would empower her for the rest of her life.

The independence that comes from the insulin pump is invaluable. When I discovered that the pump's inventor, Al Mann, was celebrating his seventy-fifth birthday, I wanted to give him something that would signify my respect, admiration, and gratitude. His invention has had such a huge impact on my life, giving me a degree of freedom I never thought possible, that I wanted to pay him back in some small way. I decided to give Mr. Mann a special photo along with one of the large stones from my crown. Although it pales in comparison to what he has given me, it is a recognition of the fact that I would not have been Miss America had it not been for his remarkable invention.

You can imagine how I felt when I received a personal note from Al Mann saying, "It is we who are grateful to be your friend and ally.... You are a role model that sets a high standard." In my book, *he* is the role model. Al also told *Business Week* that his most memorable business moment was when I won the Miss America pageant while wearing the insulin pump that he invented. But it was his invention that made me healthy, confident, and ready for the strenuous activities and demanding schedule of Miss America.

One incident during my time as Miss America made me realize how lucky I am in this respect. Soon after being crowned, I attended the Promise Ball in New York City, an annual charity for the benefit of diabetes research. Among the many celebrity guests in attendance was Mary Tyler Moore, someone I had long respected and admired—all the more so since I was diagnosed with the same disease that she has been struggling with valiantly for years. She was so quiet and withdrawn that I wondered if I'd somehow offended her. But when she went on stage and couldn't read her speech (her husband had to read it for her), I realized that diabetes had her down. It was sad, but at the same time touching to see how attentive her husband was. I couldn't help but think that I would be lucky to be married to someone so caring. That incident, however, made me more determined than ever to do everything I could to keep my disease under control and fight for a cure.

Until we find that cure, education remains one of the biggest priorities. I am determined—and I charge you—to help educators and child care providers to better understand diabetes so that the children in their care never go undetected, and to recognize, encourage, and support their students living with the challenges of diabetes every day. If you're the parent of a diabetic child, you can write your legislators asking for support. You can educate your child's teachers and friends. You can actively pursue medical research and assist funding for that research. But most important, you must understand your children and help them lead normal lives.

STAYING ON MESSAGE: TAKING IT TO THE WORLD

Diabetes, of course, is not limited to just the United States. Worldwide, over 150 million people now have diabetes, a number expected to double in the next quarter of a century. The largest growth is expected in developing countries, where proper treatment is often lacking. I remember a rare day during my time as Miss America when I was able to watch the evening news; ironically, a report was on about refugees in Chechnya dying because of a lack of insulin. Immediately, I got on the phone and tried to order some to donate overseas. I was told that this was impossible because there was insulin over there already, sitting in warehouses, being kept from the people because of bureaucratic red tape. How could any government, even during civil conflict, allow this to happen? I knew then that my efforts on behalf of those with diabetes could not be limited to the United States.

My international journey has taken me through Europe, Japan, and Mexico. To date, I have visited fifteen countries; I plan to visit many more. There is a lot of work to be done, and I can encourage others to join the cause.

I was giving my first international speech at the European Association for the Study of Diabetes Convention on Diabetes in Brussels, Belgium, when I learned what an impact even a former Miss America could have. My dear friend Susan Richmond was my traveling companion—the first "friend" that I had travel with me. During my speech, I became worried that I wasn't connecting with the audience. They weren't reacting emotionally to my presentation. I'd never had that problem in the United States. So, for the Q & A session, I moved to the floor to communicate more effectively. After about twenty minutes, the master of ceremonies closed the session. Immediately, the crowd that had been so passive rushed forward and trampled each other to get to me. It was so fast that I couldn't move out of the way. They weren't rushing me out of violence—they all wanted to touch me, to get me to sign things for them, just to see me up close. But they were pressing so much that I fell back onto the stage. The crowd had even pinned the guards that were assigned to me to the back wall. Soon, the bodyguard got onto the stage, grabbed my arms, and lifted me up. Then people poured onto the stage. The guards, Susan, and my sponsors—who had finally freed themselves—grabbed my arms and pulled me through the crowd and out to a car for safety. My friend Susan was stunned. No one knew what type of reception we would have, but no one expected this! (Would you believe my corporate clients hesitated to have me at the conference in Belgium for fear of people not being interested in Miss America?) After being mobbed again in China and Japan, I realized that being Miss America could truly have a global impact.

Now I travel not only across the United States but all over the world. Increasing diabetes awareness worldwide will save the lives of countless people. Who knows? The cure may be just around the corner, and it may be discovered by someone in a foreign land who is inspired by my words. But whatever the future holds, I will continue spreading the word—and hoping for a cure.

Chapter 11
CONTROL YOUR DIABETES FOR LIFE

When I was first diagnosed with diabetes I was devastated. I thought I was going to be controlled by diabetes for the rest of my life. It was the diabetes that dictated when I got up and when I went to bed, what I could eat and when I could eat it. I was living in fear of my blood glucose monitor. I'd see a high number and be afraid to test again. I thought the disease was my fault. Then one day I crossed a bridge—I began to realize that the more I tested, the more control I had. I realized if I didn't know what my blood sugar was, I couldn't control my disease. Once I realized that—well, I'm not going to say it's been a cakewalk—but it has helped me to really take control of the situation and of my personal care.

If you have diabetes or think you might, it is extremely important to know how to care for yourself properly and recognize the warning signs of the disease and its complications.

As I've said before, knowledge is the best weapon when fighting diabetes. A good understanding of your needs will help you to make informed decisions about your care. A thorough grasp of the facts concerning diabetes is vital not only for those who have the disease themselves but for those whom you love who have diabetes; you can make a big difference in the physical and emotional well-being of others.

EARLY DETECTION IS CRUCIAL

Diabetes isn't easy to live with, but letting it go undiagnosed is much, much worse. In addition to feeling just awful, you are putting yourself at risk for a long list of unpleasant and life-threatening complications. Being able to recognize the symptoms—in both yourself or in someone you love—could mean the difference between life and death.

For about a year before I was diagnosed, I experienced symptoms that might have given me clues to my condition had I known how to read them. But I was ignorant. I looked at each symptom individually and explained it away. It could have been a fatal mistake.

Do not be afraid to ask your doctor about unusual symptoms. Although you may be afraid that your concern is silly, remember that the life you save may be your own—or that of someone you love. In my travels as Miss America, I met many children who were diagnosed early because they had parents who knew the signs of diabetes or who just happened to notice something unusual about their child. One of the most amazing stories I heard was that of a baby who was diagnosed because of dirty diapers. This baby's mom had noticed that ants were always attracted to her baby's dirty diapers, and she wondered why. Ants hadn't been attracted to her other children's diapers.

Her curiosity led her to take an ant-infested diaper bag to the doctor. He immediately recognized that glucose in the baby's urine was attracting the ants, and he knew the baby needed to be tested for diabetes. If that mom hadn't been paying attention and asking questions, her child's diabetes might have gone unchecked for years.

Stories like this one show how important—and easy—it is to be aware of the signs. A little bit of knowledge can mean a great deal of difference for you or for the ones you love. That's why I encourage everyone, but especially parents, to learn the early signs of diabetes.

WHAT IS DIABETES?

We all know that we have to eat to fuel our bodies. When we eat, sugar is carried through our blood and is delivered to cells as fuel, giving us the energy needed to stay alive. In most people, all of this happens without any complications. Healthy people don't have to give a second thought to the levels of glucose in their blood or how well their cells are being fueled, because everything is working properly. But for a person with diabetes, this system has broken down.

There are two major types of diabetes. They have some subtle differences, but they have one crucial thing in common. In both Type I and Type II diabetes, your body has little or no ability to move glucose out of your blood and into your cells to fuel them. Also, both Type I and Type II, when left untreated, can be deadly.

TYPE I

Type I, also known as juvenile diabetes, is caused when the body, for reasons that doctors don't yet understand, destroys insulin-producing cells in the pancreas, an organ that helps you digest food. With Type I diabetes, the body stops making insulin—the hormone that helps keep the amount of sugar in the blood at a normal level. If your body doesn't make enough insulin, you end up with too much sugar in your blood and you feel awful. Symptoms can include dizziness, tiredness, and feeling grouchy. Common early warning signs of Type I diabetes include feelings of extreme thirst and needing to urinate a lot. Other symptoms may include ravenous hunger, unusual weight loss, fatigue, and blurry vision and frequent yeast infections. The symptoms of this form of diabetes often develop quickly, sometimes after an illness such as measles or mumps. This type is usually diagnosed in people under the age of thirty and often in children and teens. People with Type I diabetes must take insulin every day to stay alive. Although Type I diabetes can be treated with lifelong doses of insulin, there is no cure. There are over 1 million Americans with this form of diabetes.

TYPE II

Type II diabetes, the type that affects approximately 95 percent of the more than sixteen million people with diabetes in this country, is usually diagnosed in adults over forty. Half of all new cases of Type II diabetes occur in adults over fifty-five. But it is becoming more common in young people due to bad diet and sedentary lifestyle. Type II diabetes is a metabolic disorder—people with this form of diabetes do produce insulin, but their bodies' cells have become insulin resistant and, therefore, can't use it properly. As a result, glucose just accumulates in their blood and can't provide fuel to the cells.

Unlike Type I, Type II is often associated with being overweight or obese. Some Type II diabetics must take insulin, but many cases can be controlled through oral medications, diet, exercise, and weight loss.

Symptoms of Type II diabetes include those described for Type I, but also frequent infections, cuts and bruises that are slow to heal, tingling and numbness in hands and feet, and recurring infections of the skin, gums, or bladder. But part of the reason that close to one-third of the people with diabetes don't know that they have the disease is that you can have it and have no symptoms at all.

GESTATIONAL DIABETES

Gestational diabetes is more rare than the other forms of diabetes. Cases of gestational diabetes occur when pregnant women become insulin resistant. Typically, gestational diabetes only lasts for the duration of the pregnancy, but studies show that 40 percent of the women who experience gestational diabetes during a pregnancy go on to develop Type II within fifteen years. There are about 135,000 cases of this form of diabetes each year in this country.

Since gestational diabetes occurs in women with no previous history of the disease, all pregnant women should be tested for it between their twenty-fourth and twenty-eighth week of pregnancy. Obese women are particularly at risk, but everyone should be tested. Keeping your weight down, eating healthfully, and getting regular exercise may also help to prevent pregnancy-related insulin resistance.

WHO IS AT RISK?

While scientists don't know the exact causes of diabetes, we do know some of the risk factors for the disease. Type I diabetes is a little more mysterious than Type II. We do know that most people diagnosed with Type I diabetes are Caucasian and under the age of thirty. Family history also plays a role—we do know that Type I diabetes tends to run in families—that is to say, it is common for someone with diabetes to have a sibling with the disease. Strangely, though, most children of people with diabetes do *not* contract the disease; it can skip generations. In my case, and in the case of many others, family history was apparently not a factor. But because diabetes in the past was often undiagnosed—this is still, as I've said, an enormous problem—there are millions of people who *might* have a family history of diabetes without even knowing it.

Type I diabetes has many of the signs of being an autoimmune disorder—it kills off the beta cells in the pancreas that manufacture insulin. Because many cases of Type I appear after viral infections, scientists believe that the body might be mistaking these cells for similar-looking germs or viruses and respond by killing them off.

Type II diabetes, the more common form of the disease, also tends to run in families and usually appears in people over the age of thirty. Cases of Type II and gestational diabetes are especially common among Native Americans, African Americans, and Hispanics.

The most common trigger for Type II is obesity. Anyone whose body mass is 20 percent higher than is recommended for his or her height and weight is at high risk for Type II diabetes. Individuals who are significantly overweight or live a sedentary lifestyle can greatly reduce their risk with regular exercise and good dietary habits. Certain types of blood pressure medications and steroids are also thought to increase the risk of diabetes. Women who have had gestational diabetes or who have had a baby weighing more than nine pounds are also at an increased risk for developing Type II diabetes.

THE COMPLICATIONS

Possible complications from diabetes include heart disease, kidney disease, nerve damage (which could lead to amputation), stroke, blindness, and eye diseases like cataracts and glaucoma. Complications associated with diabetes are among the leading causes of death in this country.

The most serious and acute complication associated with Type I diabetes is something called ketoacidosis. Approximately 1,700 people die from it a year, and in people with diabetes, it kills about nine times as many people under the age of forty-five as it does people over that age. It is something that I know well because I have suffered from it—I was suffering from ketoacidosis when I was finally taken to the hospital and diagnosed with diabetes. It is a frightening and painful ordeal.

Ketoacidosis occurs when insulin levels fall far, far below the levels that the body needs. Because glucose can't get to the cells, the body becomes starved for glucose and begins to break down fat for energy. While getting rid of fat sounds like a good thing, let me assure you that it is not! The by-product of this process leaves you severely dehydrated and your blood stream packed with poisonous acids; people suffering from ketoacidosis often end up in a coma. I've learned to live with this threat. It's not pleasant, of course, but if you know what precautions to take, it doesn't have to slow you down.

People with diabetes are also at a higher risk for cardiovascular disease. Since even the most careful people with diabetes always have more glucose in their blood than people who do not have diabetes, we are at a higher risk for arteriosclerosis—

the clogging of the coronary artery. Kidney disease and even kidney failure are among the other risks that people with diabetes face. In addition, each year every person with diabetes should see a retina specialist because diabetes is the leading cause of retinal damage, and it puts the person with diabetes at an increased risk for blindness, glaucoma, and cataracts. Diabetes can also cause nerve damage to the feet and legs—with such gruesome consequences as the need for amputation.

Do I find all of this frightening? Absolutely. I would even say that some of the complications of diabetes go beyond frightening and that they even terrify me. For me, the fear of blindness is very real. I can't conceive living in a world that I couldn't see. I don't know if I would be able to survive without the sun, the light, the beauty of nature, seeing the faces of those I hold dear. So the possibility of that is definitely threatening. I also worry about the future and becoming a mother. Because of the possible complications associated with that, I pray for my future children almost daily and ask for God's protection over my body.

TAKING CHARGE: THE GOOD NEWS

If you think you might have diabetes and you have read this far, I know what you are feeling. You may be trying to explain away your symptoms as something else; it might be just coincidence that those symptoms are the same ones that I described. You are telling yourself that there is no way you want to get tested and find out that this is what your life is going to be like. If you have diabetes—and especially if you are newly diagnosed—I know exactly what you are thinking, because I have been there. You may think your life is over. You might be angry. You want to know why and you feel hopeless. I know because that was how I felt, too. Remember, I am the one who drank an entire two-liter bottle of Coke when I was told I might have diabetes because I was so angry that I didn't care if I lived or died. It's natural for you to be angry and confused for a while, but then it's time to move on.

Although there is no cure for diabetes right now, the good news is that it can be controlled, and controlling diabetes makes a big difference. When you keep your blood sugar levels in the normal range, you feel better, you have more energy, and you have the peace of mind that comes from knowing you are lowering your chances of serious complications. It is not easy to manage diabetes. Pricking your fingers several times a day to check your blood glucose can be painful and inconvenient. But it's taking charge. You have to choose healthy foods in the right amounts, try to indulge in regular physical activity, and take your diabetes medicine or insulin as prescribed. You have to make some sacrifices, but the payoff is well worth it: control your diabetes so you'll be around for your family, for your friends—for life. And the sooner you get started, the better off you will be.

HOW I TOOK CONTROL

Because I have Type I diabetes, I need insulin every day—it is my lifeline. When I was first diagnosed, I had to give myself many insulin shots a day, and I had a really hard time managing my blood glucose levels. My diabetes control was erratic, at best. In college, and then in graduate school, I was trying hard, but I just couldn't seem to control my condition. I desperately wanted to regain my freedom—and my life. I got them back with the insulin pump.

At first the pump was scary, but I learned to trust it. I could exercise with it. I could sleep soundly, without having to get up in the middle of the night to inject myself with insulin. I was finally able to tailor my diabetes care to my life, not the other way around. I felt the insulin pump made me a real person again.

HOW THE PUMP WORKS

Insulin pumps are little computerized devices about the size of an average pager that you can wear on your belt or in your pocket. The pump delivers a steady, measured dose of insulin through a flexible plastic tube called a cannula, which attaches to a fine tube called an infusion set—which is a catheter that delivers insulin from the pump to the body. You have to use a needle to insert the cannula into the skin (I use my abdomen or my hips), then you remove the needle and tape the cannula in place. In the middle of the infusion set is a quick release button that separates the pump from the cannula so that you can remove it when you take a shower, exercise vigorously, or when you need a break. Every few days you have to refill the pump with insulin and change the site on your body where you insert the cannula.

Insulin pumps can withstand a fair amount of abuse. I have had every imaginable accident with mine. I have dropped it, knocked it, gotten it caught around doorknobs, swung it off the sofa, smashed it into the coffee table, and even dropped it in the toilet. Some pumps are even waterproof—so you can swim and shower with them. That would have been a useful feature when mine went in the toilet!

Even while using the pump, you have to check your blood glucose several times a day. One of the best features of the pump is that it allows you to control the dosage of insulin based on your body's needs. The pump releases small doses of insulin continuously and can be programmed to deliver precise doses for different times of the day, mimicking the body's normal insulin releases. With the touch of a button, however, you can also give yourself the extra surge of insulin you may need when you eat or exercise.

LEARNING TO STAY HEALTHY

Though keeping your blood glucose under control is crucial, there are some other really important aspects to the care of a person with diabetes. One of those aspects is exercise. Regular exercise is imperative for a person with diabetes because it actually helps with your blood sugars.

The important thing about exercise is to take advantage of the time you have to do *something*, every day. If you're not always on the road, set an exercise schedule and stick to it. A dirty little secret to exercise programs and videos is that they're essentially all the same. The trick doesn't lie in some gimmick. All you have to do is get on your feet and do it. Jumping jacks, jumping rope, walking, jogging, lifting weights (any kind of weights will do), push ups, lunges, whatever you like, as long as you get about thirty minutes of a cardiovascular workout a day and spend at least ten minutes a day on stretching and doing strength exercises. As Miss America, I even carried a jump rope in my suitcase for this purpose; I still feel sorry for the people sleeping in the room beneath me in all those hotels I stayed in.

Maintaining an exercise schedule was one of the hardest things for me in the year I was on the road as Miss America (although the travel has slowed down a bit, it's still hard). The constant traveling was exhausting, and when each day was over, I had no desire to exercise. Because I had only one day off a month, I had to be creative. I treated airports as if they were gyms. I started wearing tennis shoes when I traveled so that I could use the "down time" in airport terminals to do some brisk walking. I would do lunges and jumping jacks on the jet way, stretches in the plane, and there was always lots of room in the terminals to speed walk. I was, in fact, a walking exercise video. I'm sure some people thought it looked a bit strange, but with the stress of constant travel, I needed to exercise to help keep my blood sugars at a healthy level.

EATING WELL

Obviously, to stay healthy, you need to eat well. The most important thing is balance. It is important to control portion size—while it is easy to eat right, it is sometimes difficult to eat the right amounts. For instance, many of us like carbohydrates a lot more than we like protein. So, we just have to be careful about what we eat.

Giving up some of your favorite foods is tough; the hardest thing for me to give up was drinking Coke! Sometimes you will struggle with that desire for sweets and baked goods—I know I do. But you can have them in moderation, along with a balanced diet. Most people give little thought to the food they consume, but for a person with diabetes, each decision about food can directly affect your life and longevity.

In a perfect world, we would all be able to eat cheesecake, cherry pie, and Krispy Kreme donuts every day. But we can't. People with diabetes, especially, have to make sensible choices if we are going to have a long and healthy lives. Because it's not always easy to make those sensible choices, I recently collaborated on a cookbook called *Mr. Food's Quick & Easy Diabetic Cooking Featuring Nicole Johnson*; the recipes you'll find in it are not only for those with diabetes but for everyone concerned about eating right. There's even a recipe for cheesecake (which is, to be honest, my favorite in the book).

While traveling as Miss America and as a spokesperson for diabetes, I've found that eating regular meals is not all that simple. I have discovered that I often don't get to eat at a speaking engagement. Typically, the food is served, and it looks wonderful, but as a speaker or a guest, I find myself engrossed in preparation for my talk, hosting the dinner, performing on stage, or in constant polite conversation. On the bright side—this can be great for the waistline. I have, however, suffered many lows (low blood sugar levels) as a result of this kind of thing.

People often wonder why celebrities make demands when booking events. I now understand—I never stay at any hotel unless it has twenty-four-hour room service. Since I never get to eat at events, I always go back to my room and order dinner afterwards. I guess you could call it one of the tricks of the trade!

TAKING CONTROL OF YOUR HEART

An interesting question that is often posed to me is, "How do you cope?" The truth is that there is really no single surefire way of dealing with this condition. It is important to realize that diabetes is very different for each individual. Methods of care can vary greatly, based on physical and emotional needs. There are, however, a few basic things that have really helped my family and me cope with diabetes that I would definitely recommend to anyone facing this or any other chronic condition:

◆ *A good doctor and a good relationship with your medical team* When I was diagnosed, we found a physician whom I could trust. It is so important to have faith in your medical team and to know—deep in your heart—that your doctors and nurses are doing all they can to help you.

◆ *A support group or team*

I don't have a group that I go visit, but I consider my family and a few close friends my diabetes support group. I know that I can call them when I am feeling down or having a hard time with my diabetes control. In fact, they know me so well that they can often tell when I need them, before I ask. I know that they won't belittle me but will support and uplift me. They are capable of giving me a swift kick in the rear when I get out of line, though. I also know that I can celebrate my successes with them. That is so important.

◆ *I live my life with a lot of hope*

Each day I live with the knowledge that medical science is advancing by the hour. I've visited the labs, seen the work, and felt the dream of a cure. That constant thought is very helpful to my family and me. We make it a practice to share news articles and research information so that we can keep up with the most recent developments in diabetes research.

◆ *I use sources of inspiration to help me along the way*

When I get down, I reflect on those I know who have had diabetes for many, many years. They are my inspiration. I think about the people I have seen achieve the "50 Years with Diabetes" medal, which is awarded by the Joslin Diabetes Center and Eli Lilly. I also think about the kids that I have met who live with this every day. It helps me to remember that all over the world, we are all facing the same struggle, and we are all working toward the same goal. I know that at any given time, there are many of us testing our blood glucose levels together. We are all warriors in the same battle—if we want to win, we can't give up or let the enemy cross the lines. I also tend to think of other achievers and challenge myself with their successes. I have found great comfort in the courage of those who have suffered some of the complications of diabetes but haven't allowed it to crush their spirits. One of these heroes is Paralympic medalist Pam Fernandez, who hasn't let blindness and kidney failure stand in her way. Another is Mark Collie, the country music songwriter and singer (and semipro race car driver) who is a vocal diabetes advocate as well. Mark has been such a good friend to me and others with diabetes. He is a hero and a role model. Both Mark and Pam are definitely a source of inspiration for anyone struggling with this disease.

◆ *I rely on my faith to help me cope with my diabetes*
Prayer is a huge part of my diabetes care and control. I accept the fact that I can do nothing on my own. My faith in God's love, grace, and providence really helps pull me through. I don't know why I have diabetes but I know that I have a mission to accomplish with this condition in my life. For me, that focus and faith is essential to my peace of mind.

◆ *I play a game with my diabetes*
This often helps me to look at diabetes in a different light. I try to turn things around and make diabetes a personal competition—a game with real rewards and setbacks. For instance, I will challenge myself to two days with perfect (in my mind) blood glucose levels. If I accomplish this, I might give myself permission to have

a great desert or take a trip to the ice cream shop. (Now, mind you, I don't do this all the time, but sometimes it is good to have a sweet incentive!)

The encouraging news is this: every day scientists and doctors around the world are learning new things about this disease and are one step closer to finding a cure. The other thing to know is that, with proper treatment, a person with diabetes can live a healthy and full life with minimal complications. There is a lot to be encouraged by. Most important, we are not alone. There are well over sixteen million of us in America living with this condition each day, and the lives that these millions touch are innumerable. If we all work together, we can raise awareness and, someday soon, find a cure. In fact, we are closer now than we ever have been.

HOPE FOR THE FUTURE

Anyone who suffers from diabetes can tell you that keeping hope alive is a vital aspect of the daily battle. Looking at the known facts about the seriousness of my condition, it would be easy to become disheartened. Even with close monitoring of my blood glucose levels, there is no guarantee that the constant war my diabetes wages against my system will not take its toll.

But hope is the great equalizer. Hope is stronger than any despair. Hope—rooted in faith—gives breath to action, and the first necessary action is to take responsibility for dealing with my disease. One of the quotations that I frequently repeat to myself and others as a motivational call to action is the following (ironically, I can't remember the source): "Vision without action is only a dream. Action without vision merely passes time. But vision with action changes the world."

When people ask me how I cope, I tell them that I do it day-by-day: daily monitoring and treatment, daily prayers for faith and optimism, and daily determination to do what I can to help medical scientists find a cure. Diabetes can be devastating and difficult to live with, but it is never impossible as long as you maintain hope. I firmly believe that God gives us everything we need to face the challenges and to find solutions. We need faith and hope as much as we need insulin.

HOW FAR HAVE WE COME?

While there is never a good time to have diabetes, now is such an exciting time for this disease. Wonderful advances are being made in the search for a cure—and I am positive that within the next decade or two scientists will find one—whether through some form of gene therapy or the invention of an artificial pancreas. I feel sure that the cure for this disease is on the horizon.

I often reflect on how fortunate I am to live now, when we're enjoying such rapid progress in medical knowledge. It really gives you perspective and a deep sense of gratitude to realize that until quite recently, people with diabetes had no chance for a normal life or even an average life span. It is a well-documented fact that before 1922, when insulin was first made available, babies of mothers with diabetes simply did not survive. Today, a woman with diabetes has about the same chance of delivering a normal healthy baby as a woman who does not have diabetes, as long as she keeps tight control on her blood glucose during pregnancy. And fewer than 6 percent of parents with Type I diabetes pass their condition onto their children. This is good news for me. As I have said, being a mother is a deep and heartfelt desire, but I want to be sure that

I give my future children every opportunity to live long and healthy lives. While I am completely open to adopting children and have been discouraged by some about becoming pregnant, I also know that every day doctors and scientists are learning more about this disease and how it affects expectant mothers and their babies. If I do decide to have children, I know that it will be a team effort to ensure that they are healthy, but I continue to be encouraged by the current research and what the future holds.

We are truly fortunate to live in this day and age. Not long ago, medicine was in such a primitive state of development that effective treatment—not to mention a cure—for diabetes was inconceivable. People had no alternative other than to suffer from the complications of their undiagnosed disease and, in most cases, eventually to succumb to it. We have come so far that while I sometimes worry about how long it will take to find a cure, I gain strength from knowing that scientific research into the causes and possible cures of diabetes is moving forward literally daily. Today we are further along in the fight against diabetes than we were yesterday. Tomorrow we'll be closer still. Science itself is the cure for despair—and complacency.

ONE STEP CLOSER TO A CURE

One of the most promising possibilities of a cure for Type I diabetes is called islet cell transplantation. Islet cells are the cells in the pancreas that produce insulin—the very cells that the body seems to attack and destroy in Type I diabetes. Once these cells are destroyed, the body can't produce insulin.

Unfortunately, while some 270 transplants of islet cells have been attempted since 1989, in only 8 percent of these procedures have the new cells been accepted and been able to restore the body's ability to produce insulin. The good news, though, is that a medical team at the University of Alberta Hospital in Edmonton, Canada, has recently made significant breakthroughs in several areas. The scientists have learned how to better harvest the cells and have figured out how many of these are needed to achieve "insulin independence." They are also devising new and more sophisticated antirejection drugs that will make this procedure safer and more effective. As Alberta Foundation executive director JoAnne Langer said of the new breakthrough, "It is not a cure, but we are a step closer. It is the most hope for people with diabetes that they've heard in years."

This groundbreaking research was made possible by a small nonprofit outfit, the Alberta Foundation for Diabetes Research, which funded the team's work through charity golf tournaments and auctions—through money that came from people like you and me. That donations from private individuals led to such a major step towards finding a cure is an inspiration for all of us who raise money for diabetes research. Every research team we can support raises the odds of discovering a cure. Every dollar does count.

And this isn't just laboratory theory. Islet cell transplants are already saving lives. A man named Byron Best is living proof that such transplants can work. He was one of the first successful recipients of this procedure in 1999. At fifty-five, he had been suffering from sudden blackouts for years. Blackouts come from sudden plunges of blood glucose levels—what I call a low—which are typical of both types of diabetes. For Byron, as for many others, insulin injections just weren't enough. And for Byron, the result of a blackout was almost fatal, not because of a complication, but because of timing.

His last blackout before his surgery happened while he was riding his motorcycle. There was a serious accident, and he was lucky to survive. The silver lining, though, was that this accident led to an islet cell transplant following the new method innovated by the Edmonton team. It worked. Today, Byron no longer needs daily injections of insulin.

Byron's story is another example of how hope sustains people with diabetes. Even in the worst days of his diabetes, he never lost hope for a cure. "There's always a hope, there's always a glimmer, even if the technology is not there yet," he said last year. "The only thing that keeps you going, that keeps you sane, is the hope that somebody's got to come up with a solution to this."

There is still a long way to go. Islet cell transplants are not yet the cure we're looking for. For the vast majority of people with Type I diabetes, the possible complications or side effects of antirejection drugs make the procedure too risky. The dangers still outweigh the benefits except in extreme cases. Moreover, at its present stage of development, the cost of the operation is prohibitively expensive for most people. In the United States, where health insurance rarely pays for experimental treatments, islet cell transplants can cost anywhere between $50,000 and $100,000. Most people don't earn that much in a year.

Another very hopeful research development was first reported just last year. Scientists at Yonsei University Medical School in Seoul, Korea, were actually able to use gene therapy to turn the livers of rodents into insulin factories that regulated blood sugar, just like the pancreas is supposed to do. Although the insulin production of the treated rodents was only 20 to 40 percent of the normal rate, it was enough to control blood glucose. While still in its preliminary stages, this research has the potential to revolutionize the current approach to treatment.

A MORAL DILEMMA

Genetic research holds promise for people suffering from Type II diabetes, too. In September 1999, a team of researchers in San Francisco and Italy announced that they had identified the gene that causes insulin resistance. This was a huge discovery and evidence that, for diabetes to be cured rather than just managed, genetic research will play a big role. It also raises big questions, the most difficult of which is the issue of stem cell research.

Although stem cell research is still in preliminary stages, many scientists think it has great potential for helping to find a cure. But most proponents of stem cell research advocate experimenting on the stem cells taken from aborted fetuses. To be useful, the cells must be taken from fetuses that are either newly aborted or frozen. In either case, both techniques raise some serious moral questions—and they are certainly morally unacceptable if they create a commercial market for selling fetal parts.

I have strong feelings about the moral implications of abortion, and these are guided by my abiding belief in the value and sanctity of all human life, a belief that has its roots in my Christian faith. I know that every life is a precious gift from God. The value of each human person doesn't depend on money, how her organs could be used, whether she is "wanted" or "unwanted," or whether she is genetically perfect or genetically flawed. As someone who has Type I diabetes, a disease that's genetic in origin, I'm particularly sensitive to this type of language. Physical adversity is no reason to make the judgment that a life is not worth living.

From my understanding of the issue, however, there do seem to be conditions under which stem cell research may not be objectionable (such as using the stem cells of living adults or those from umbilical cord tissue), but it remains to be seen whether these are viable methods. So here, as is the case in so many aspects of research, we need to remain optimistic but not lose our sense of morality. I desperately want to find a cure for this disease, but I don't want it at the expense of others or because I have compromised my morals. I believe that it is possible to find a cure without such a compromise—and that the answer to our hopes is just around the corner.

One of the things that medical science teaches us is that learning about diabetes, or any disease, is a lifelong process. Scientists are still learning so much. Obviously, when I was first diagnosed with diabetes, I had a long way to go and many lessons to learn. But that journey of learning—of overcoming the pain, humiliation, sickness, and personal setbacks, and of finding a scheme, or a plan, that explains what has happened in my life—has made me a much better person, so much so that I can even thank God for my disease. As Supreme Court justice Clarence Thomas said, "It takes a person with a mission to succeed." Diabetes gave me a mission. And when I look in the smiling eyes of a child, when I see us getting closer to a cure for this disease, I feel that I am on the road to success.

Chapter 12

GIVING YOUR BEST

I would not be the person I am today had I not been diagnosed with diabetes. It has made me realize the power that comes from fighting for what you believe in and facing up to adversity. I have gained perspective on what is truly important and developed strength of character that I never possessed before.

I guess you could say that my personal philosophy comes down to one simple, but profound, idea: giving your best. It's really impossible for any of us to do more than that. When I was younger, I thought that giving your best meant accepting nothing less than perfection. Now, I know that giving your best is a choice you make despite your imperfections. In order to give all that you have, you first have to accept the cards that you have been dealt. You have to accept yourself as you are— with all of your limitations, flaws, and constraints. Don't allow yourself to give in to useless wishful thinking: if only I could change this or that, if only I were in a different situation, *then* I would be able to achieve my dreams. No, you wouldn't, because you've already adopted the attitude of the defeated. As a wise man once said, "Success is a state of mind. If you want success, start thinking of yourself as a success." It isn't until you accept yourself as you are and see your situation as it is that you can begin to figure out how to get past the obstacles in your life. If you refuse to see the obstacle, you will end up running right into it.

But no one can do this on their own. Although an attitude of faith and hope is essential, I really believe that it would be impossible to find the strength to fight any battle without the support of friends and family. Giving your best is only possible if you have people around you who believe in you. Personally, I know that I couldn't do it without my family. In many ways, diabetes has made me more aware of my need for others: a need to talk things out (even to vent, sometimes), a need to share, to be reassured, and to consult with others about the course I plan to take. In these things, my friends and family have been indispensable. If I didn't have them, I really doubt whether I could survive, much less give my best.

I don't want to give the impression that I'm always a tower of strength. I continually seek affirmation, guidance, and encouragement—especially from the hard-won wisdom of people who have struggled and come out on top. There's a quote that I particularly cherish from the late football coach Vince Lombardi: "The greatest accomplishment is not in never falling, but in rising again after you fall." How true this is! Giving in to discouragement after failure or frustration is something I try to avoid. Not that I'm always successful. There was even a time when the frustration and pain of my diabetes took me into a dark night of the soul. Thank God for those who helped me through this time when my thoughts and emotions were so full of despair. Without the support of family and friends who prayed for and with me during that time, I wouldn't have been able to pull through.

From time to time, I still have ups and downs. I struggle to stay on top of those areas of my life where I feel least secure. On some days, I worry about my future with diabetes and I just sit and cry. It is hard to cope with the fact that my life span could be cut short by ten to fifteen years because of this condition. Although I know that the majority of complications can be prevented with good care and control, I also know that some people fall prey to complications no matter what they do. Sometimes I am afraid that this will happen to me.

I also struggle against the tendency to worry too much about what others think of me. I have had to learn through hard experience that you can't please everyone, and I know you shouldn't even try. I do want people to like me and to be pleased with my work, but I know this won't always be the case. In my quest in the past for acceptance—and even as Miss America—I hid a lot about my diabetes and myself. That sometimes led to big problems. As I get older, I realize that sharing these things is essential. Keeping everything bottled up is a recipe for trouble.

There have also been new challenges to face. During my year as Miss America, my parents separated, and in 2001 they divorced. Even in my late twenties, this is still a difficult reality to accept. Divorce affects children at any age. It causes you to question the reality of the life you grew up in and your own ability to commit to and succeed in relationships. I love both my parents, but their divorce hurts me. Their separation was particularly difficult to deal with while traveling across the country as Miss America—wondering what people would think, worrying about how it was going to affect my brother, wishing I could be there, at home.

But I always return to two truths that put all the difficulties in perspective: first, everything happens for a reason, and second, God never gives you more than you can bear. You can always gain something from the challenges you face, and if you turn to God for help, He will always pull you through. Even if I don't understand today why certain things have to happen the way they do, tomorrow I may see why they were blessings in disguise. And regardless of whether I understand it or not, it will all work out for the best. I know that worrying about an unknown future doesn't do any good, and worrying about a current obstacle doesn't help the situation. I've found that it's important to pray and entrust everything to God. I don't have all of the answers yet, but I know that He is taking care of me and that He has given me a job here on earth. And when I apply myself to the mission He has given me, when I give my best each day, I feel most at peace.

In the meantime, I try to practice what I preach; I try to live by the rules that I taught to kids all across the country, when I was traveling as Miss America, adapted, of course, to someone who's a bit older:

◆ *Wake up, show up, and pay attention*
This rule comes from a friend I know in the air force, Lieutenant Commander Drew Brown. In order to give your best, you have to be fully engaged in what you are doing. You have to be on time, be prepared for what you're doing, and focus completely on the task at hand, not allowing yourself to get sidetracked. A lot of promising beginnings come to nothing due to lack of attention and focus.

◆ *Love something, particularly yourself*

We are all made to love. Unless we love by giving ourselves to others—God, family, friends—we are unfulfilled. But before you can give yourself, you have to love yourself, not in a narcissistic, self-centered way, but simply in the sense of recognizing that the talents, qualities, and opportunities that you've been given are unique. And that they are given to you for a reason. If you value what you've been given, if you value who you are, you're more likely to use your talents generously for the benefit of others.

◆ *If you refuse to give up, you cannot fail*

Perseverance: as long as you continue to pursue a goal, it is still within your reach. If you keep moving ahead, apparent failures are only temporary setbacks. This truth really helps me not to give in to discouragement, and to get up and begin again after a fall.

The song that I performed in the Miss America pageant in Atlantic City the year I won the crown actually summarizes a lot of these themes. It's called "That's Life," and it was made famous by Frank Sinatra, although I learned it from a videotape of another girl in the Miss Virginia pageant ten years before I competed. As I learned the words and the tune by watching the tape, I fell in love with the song. It seemed to echo my own thoughts and feelings about my life and my struggle with diabetes...

That's life, that's what the people say, ridin' high in April, shot down in May

Before I was diagnosed with diabetes, I was frequently told things like "you're really the Miss America type" and "you have a great future in pageant competition." After people became aware that I had diabetes, it was a different story. "You'll never be able to win because you don't fit the Barbie doll image of Miss America" was a typical comment. Or "Be realistic: you won't be able to handle the stress with your condition." If you base your view of what you can achieve on what you hear from others rather than on your own inner conviction, you'll never achieve your dreams.

I know I'm gonna change that tune, 'cause I'll be back on top in June

June was the month of the Miss Virginia pageant, and I vowed to myself that I would prove all the naysayers wrong. I was simply not going to accept advice from others, however well intentioned, telling me that my diabetes would keep me from achieving my dreams. Achievement in this case didn't necessarily mean winning; it was an achievement just to be there, doing the best I could. Of course, winning, too, was a great achievement, but it's not what I expected.

Some people get their kicks steppin' on dreams, but I won't let life get me down, 'cause this big old world just keeps goin' around

Ever since I was diagnosed with diabetes, I've been told that certain things are impossible. I've been told that I couldn't graduate from college; that I couldn't become a television journalist; that I couldn't become Miss America. Some people like to be negative, but you can't let that negativity dictate what you do. You can't let it present an insuperable obstacle to the healthy ambition you have within you to make your dreams reality. If you refuse to give up, you'll be a winner in the end.

Each time I find myself flat on my face, I pick myself up and get back in the race

I competed in the Miss America program for six years; I had been beaten many times. But I kept picking myself up and getting back in the race. There's a verse in Philippians that says if you finish the race, God will help you.

At every stage of competing for the title of Miss America, my platform of diabetes awareness was my inspiration; it was the mission I had been entrusted with that gave me the determination I needed to pick myself up and keep going. I think that everyone needs a real sense of purpose in life to be able to keep up the effort of giving her best, day in and day out. I hope that as Miss America, and as a spokesperson for those with diabetes, I've been able to help inspire people—both those suffering from my disease, as well as those who don't but now understand a little more clearly what is at stake in this battle. Everybody's searching for something—something to believe in, that will nurture self-confidence and purpose. If I've been able to provide that to only a few, it's been worth the effort.

As for me, one of the things I take most pride in is the fact that each time I won a major pageant—both in the Miss Virginia and the Miss America competitions—I was captured on live television saying, "Thank you, Jesus." He's the one who deserves the credit for my successes and to whom I owe a debt that I can't begin to repay. He is the reason why I am who I am, and the reason why I have achieved what I have achieved. To be able to declare that on national television is a great blessing in itself.

Just recently, I've been fortunate enough to become friends with Congressman Randy Forbes of Virginia. The first time we met, as we talked about his political prospects and my work in raising diabetes awareness and finding a cure, I recognized that there was something special about this man. Unlike many who are prominent in the public eye, Randy is not afraid of speaking the truth with boldness and clarity, and calling them as he sees them. He is one of my true role models, not least because he has shown me that you don't have to change who you are or your beliefs for the sake of being popular—even if you are a politician.

At that first meeting, he also gave me something which has been a huge influence on my life ever since, a little book called *The Prayer of Jabez: Breaking Through to the Blessed Life.* It contains reflections on a simple prayer found in the Old Testament book of Chronicles: "Oh, that You would bless me indeed, and enlarge my territory, that Your hand would be with me, and that You would keep me from evil, that I may not cause pain." The lesson that author Bruce Wilkinson draws from this ancient prayer is simple: *You have not because you ask not.* In other words, only if you are persistent in asking God for His grace will you be able to find the determination and energy to overcome the obstacles you encounter in life. As he handed me the book, Randy told me that he hoped I would continue to keep asking for blessings, no matter what obstacle might come my way.

In my own life, I've found that God always answers prayers, but not always in the way you expect. I always knew that God had a mission for me in the world; I just didn't understand what it was until I was diagnosed with diabetes. Now I have more determination and purpose than ever before. But living with diabetes hasn't always been easy for me. For many months, I struggled with fear, denial, anger, and depression— all reactions to the shock of being diagnosed with a life-threatening disease that, as yet, has no cure. I felt trapped. I felt my life was being stolen from me. But one day, I found the spirit of determination deep within me, the determination to educate myself and others about my disease, to do all I could to conquer it and help other diabetics conquer it. In fact, I remember the exact moment when the transformation—from defeated, bitter victim of life, to optimistic fighter, determined to pursue my dreams—began. I was talking with my parents after the severe reaction I had in 1997 about my future prospects. I mentioned all the advice I had received to quit school, cut back on my activity, give up my dream of becoming Miss America, and adopt a more "realistic" approach to my goals in life, goals that would now—of necessity—have to be curtailed. Suddenly, I became irate, stomping the ground and making a fist, telling them that if anyone had a reason to compete, I did. I had a message to give. I had a purpose. People needed to know about diabetes, that it didn't have to stop them from anything, even if people told them otherwise.

In retrospect, it was at that moment that I found my focus. I stopped brooding, started on a course to educate people about diabetes, and determined then and there to take another try at becoming Miss Virginia, whatever the outcome.

Today, I often tell the young people I meet the story of how I nearly gave up because of my diabetes, and I warn them, "Don't ever let anyone tell you that you can't do something because you have diabetes. Don't ever let it stop you from becoming anything you want to be—lawyer, writer, teacher, scientist, or even Miss America."

It's a story I'm still living out.

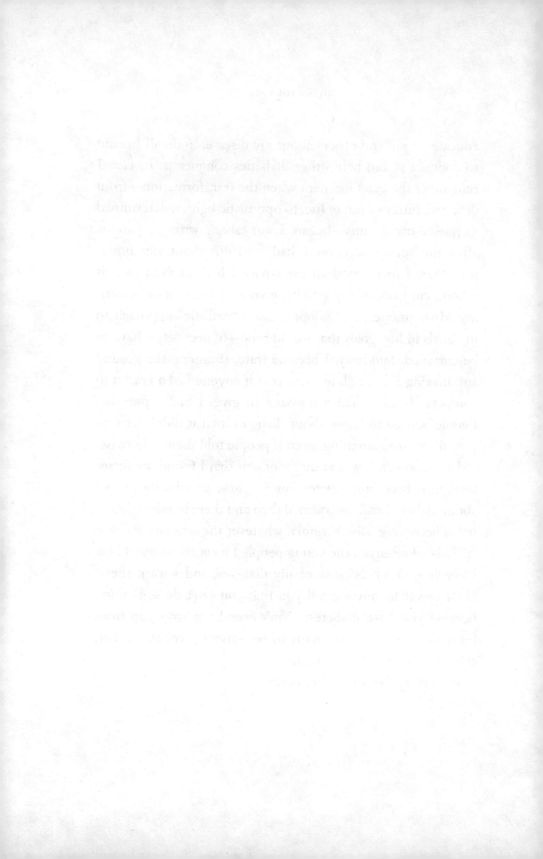

Appendix A
MY DAILY ROUTINE OF DIABETES CARE, DIET, AND EXERCISE

*I*n terms of my diabetes care, I test my glucose anywhere between six and ten times a day. I try to stay on top of my glucose levels so that I never get too far outside of my target range. I do have to say, though, that my glucose levels are far from perfect. I average about a 7.0 A1c level; I am doing everything I can to get into the 6.0 range. I typically infuse anywhere from 30 to 40 units of insulin a day into my body by means of my insulin pump.

Diabetes care is different for each individual, so please use this guide as just that—a guide. My diabetes is different from your own or that of your loved ones. It is important to seek advice from your personal medical professional to determine what treatment is best for you.

Here's a rough idea of my daily routine:

7:00 A.M.

I get up. I usually eat Fiber One cereal or oatmeal and raisins sprinkled with Equal artificial sweetener. I then go and take a brisk walk or make a trip to the gym. If I go to the gym, I walk on the treadmill or use the Elliptical machine for about a half-hour and then do strength training for another 20 to 30 minutes.

12 NOON–1:30 P.M.

I typically eat lunch around this time. My lunches consist of anything from fruit salad to yogurt and some fruit or a light sandwich. (I do love to make PB&J sandwiches or peanut butter and banana sandwiches on occasion.) After lunch, I get back to work.

4:00 P.M.

This is when the munchies set in for me. I sometimes grab a handful of raisins or some crackers to ease the need/desire for food. I also always monitor my glucose during this time of the day to make sure that I am not slumping too low.

6:00–9:00 P.M.

I usually eat dinner somewhere in this time frame; it all depends on what my schedule permits. Dinner typically consists of chicken and veggies—and of course some carbs. I love to make entrées from the cookbook I collaborated on, *Mr. Food's Quick & Easy Diabetic Cooking*. Some of my favorites for dinner are Mediterranean Chicken, Bottomless Chicken Pot Pie, Johnson's Pasta-Rama, and Golden Crab Cakes. Sometimes, if I am at home, I go for a walk after dinner to relax and work off some of those calories. Many times, though, I go right back to work.

In a typical day, I spend anywhere from two to four hours on the computer, about two hours on the phone, and the rest of my time working on various projects. I confess to being a news junkie (I did study journalism in graduate school, after all), so I never go to bed without getting my fill of current events and hot topics.

Appendix B
A DIABETES RESOURCE GUIDE

*K*nowledge is truly the best way we can equip ourselves for this disease. A sense of community is also vital. We are not alone in our fight against diabetes, and it helps to know that. The Internet has become a fantastic resource for diabetics. There are numerous informative websites that can provide information on treatment research and medical product information. They also provide a sense of community through chat rooms and ways of contacting support groups in your area. You can even shop for your medications on some of them. The options are almost limitless, but some of the best are listed below.

GENERAL INFORMATION
www.cdc.gov is the official website of the Centers for Disease Control and Prevention, the primary federal agency for protecting the health and safety of Americans. In the area of the

site devoted to diabetes, you can find important information about the extent of the diabetes epidemic, a "National Diabetes Fact Sheet" (a helpful summary of fact and figures about the disease), and a comprehensive "Diabetes Surveillance Report," which is perhaps the best and most thorough primer on diabetes now available.

www.diabetes.com is part of PlanetRx.com. This is the site to go to if you want information about different devices, including insulin pumps and glucose monitors. It has a comprehensive guide to products, devices, and medications. It is also an online drugstore, so you can buy your medication through the site. In addition, it has plenty of helpful information, tips, and community chats.

www.diabetes.org is the official website of the American Diabetes Association. The site has great articles, information for the newly diagnosed, current and new information about living with diabetes, information about new technological advances, recipes, local information, bookstore, and links to *Diabetes Forecast*, the ADA's magazine. The site is also available in Spanish. The ADA's toll free number is 1 (800) DIABETES.

www.joslin.harvard.edu is the official website of the Joslin Diabetes center in Boston, MA. The center is affiliated with the Harvard medical school and is the only American medical center dedicated solely to diabetes research, treatment, and education. The site has an online library and an excellent crash course for the newly diagnosed called "The Beginner's Guide to Diabetes." You can order a free diabetes information packet from Joslin through the website or by calling 1 (800) JOSLIN1.

www.niddk.nih.gov is the website for the National Institute for Diabetes, Digestive, and Kidney Disease, part of the National Institutes of Health. The site is good for information on research developments, special congressional reports, and clinical trials of experimental therapies. The site is available in Spanish and easy-to-read versions.

CHILDREN, TEENS, AND JUVENILE DIABETES
www.childrenwithdiabetes.com is "the online community for kids, families, and adults with diabetes." This site and its sister-site, **www.diabetes123.com**, have great online stores for books, diabetes products, and even games. They also sponsor online chats with doctors, have great recipes, and the D Team, a group of health care professionals on hand to answer questions. To reach Children with Diabetes by phone, call (805) 492-6530.

www.jdrf.org is the website for the Juvenile Diabetes Research Foundation International. JDRF is the world's leading nonprofit, nongovernmental supporter of diabetes research. This site has great up-to-date links to the news stories and issues surrounding diabetes research and funding. You can also learn how to become a JDRF legislative advocate on this site. To contact JDRF, call (800) 533-CURE.

www.pumpgirls.com is where you can learn more about a remarkable group of young ladies. The Pump Girls, a group of talented teens from Southern California, met at camp and formed a singing group. They all are "pumpers" like me and they are a huge inspiration to youngsters with diabetes—and adults, too! A portion of the proceeds from their CD sales goes to the Pediatric Adolescent Diabetes Research and Education (PADRE) Foundation.

TREATMENT AND PRODUCT INFORMATION

www.adaenet.org can help you to find a diabetes educator anywhere in the country. ADAE is the American Association of Diabetes Educators and represents over 10,000 health care professionals who provide diabetes education and care. This is a must-see website for anyone trying to put together a medical support team. You can call ADAE at (312) 424-2426.

www.DiabetesManager.com is an Internet-based service providing the decision support you need to optimally control your diabetes based on your physician's prescription. The better you control your diabetes the lower your chance of complications.

www.diabeteswell.com is an online clinic with real time access to doctors and specialists. For a fee, you can use the site to track and analyze your medications, glucose levels, and general progress. The site also offers personalized action plans. You can call Diabetes Well at (800) 322-2033 for more information.

www.equal.com is the website of the nonsugar sweetener Equal, featuring a "Diabetes Education Center" which gives a brief background on diabetes risk factors, symptoms, and treatment. More importantly, the site includes a "Recipe Box" where you can find dozens of sugar-free recipes that you won't believe are sugar-free!

www.insulin-pumpers.org provides information and support for adults and children with diabetes and their families interested in insulin pump therapy. There is a special section devoted to children with diabetes and the stories about how an insulin pump has changed their lives.

www.lillydiabetes.com contains a wealth of information to help you manage your diabetes. It's a particularly good source of tips on diabetes management, and information about Eli Lilly products is also featured.

www.medicalert.org is the website for Medic Alert bracelets and necklaces. If you are in an accident or are so ill that you can't speak for yourself, these are lifesaving devices. A doctor, nurse, or EMT will recognize the emblem and know that you need special treatment. For a nominal annual fee, your medical history is kept in Medic Alert's computer system, where any medical professional can access it twenty-four hours a day. You can register online or by calling (888) 633-4298.

www.minimed.com offers all kinds of information on pump therapy, including informational packages and movies available for downloading. This, as you must know by now, is the pump that I wear. There is an online store as well as stories on other "pumpers." If you contact MiniMed at (800) MINIMED and ask for information, you can get a video hosted by yours truly.

OFF THE BEATEN PATH
http://pages.prodigy.net/dfan/dfansite/index.html is the website for the Diabetic Friends Action Network. This has a fun site for kids, but it also has a great online newsletter and a bookstore with a good selection of general information books, cookbooks, and children's books focused on diabetes.

www.diabetes-exercise.org is the site for the International Diabetic Athletes Association. IDAA has regional chapters all over the country for diabetic athletes. Find training partners or just some new friends. The website lists local contacts for chapters in your area and a calendar for upcoming races and events. You can contact IDAA at 1 (800) 898-IDAA.

Acknowledgments

John Swanston, I owe you so much. Your intelligence and compassion stun me daily. I wouldn't have been able to complete this project if it hadn't been for you. Thank you for sharing the vision—your faith helped make this dream a reality. You are my hero!

Jennifer Franklin, thank you for helping save the day. Your friendship is a precious gift.

Regnery/Lifeline Publishing, thank you for your patience and dedication to excellence.

Michelle Kang, your support, love, and friendship are a treasure. Thank you for the motivation and memories!

Bill Baker, the cover photo is gorgeous. It is amazing how you can capture my heart and put it on photo paper. Thank you for making me look beautiful!

My family, Emily, George, and Scott, you have sustained me over the years. Thank you for caring and helping me grow into the person I am. Boy, do I have great genes!

Everyone at the *American Diabetes Association*, you believed in me and have allowed me to spread my wings and fly. It is a pleasure to be associated with you.

My *JDRF* family, your commitment to research thrills my soul. Thank you for working to find OUR cure!

MiniMed, you are my lifesavers. Thank you for being there to "pump me up." My heart will always be with you—you have my dedication and eternal gratitude.

Eli Lilly, my insulin partner, thank you for believing in me and allowing me to represent you worldwide.

Joslin Diabetes Center, thank you for taking care of me. I am honored to be your chairperson of the High Hopes Fund for Kids with Diabetes and your patient.

The Miss America Organization, I will be forever indebted to you for your support and encouragement. Thank you for my education and the gift of association with you.

The Miss Virginia Organization, you are my other family! Thank you for everything—you are fabulous and I am proud to be a daughter of the Old Dominion.

My Heavenly Father, your love is so amazing. You are faithful, precious, holy, and merciful. Thank you for the greatest gift of all—**to you I give all the glory, for you made all this possible**!